Rigoberto Pérez Ramos
Efren Padrón
Andrieli D. Zdanski

Improving health care for the elderly at UBS Barrinha, Matias Olímpio

Rigoberto Pérez Ramos
Efren Padrón
Andrieli D. Zdanski

Improving health care for the elderly at UBS Barrinha, Matias Olímpio

Family Health

ScienciaScripts

Imprint

Cover image: www.ingimage.com

This book is a translation from the original published under ISBN 978-613-9-63650-1.

Publisher:
Sciencia Scripts
is a trademark of
Dodo Books Indian Ocean Ltd. and OmniScriptum S.R.L publishing group

120 High Road, East Finchley, London, N2 9ED, United Kingdom
Str. Armeneasca 28/1, office 1, Chisinau MD-2012, Republic of Moldova, Europe
Printed at: see last page
ISBN: 978-620-7-69262-0

What has to grow in the world is not discovering how it is now, but the effort of each one to discover it.

Napoleon Hill

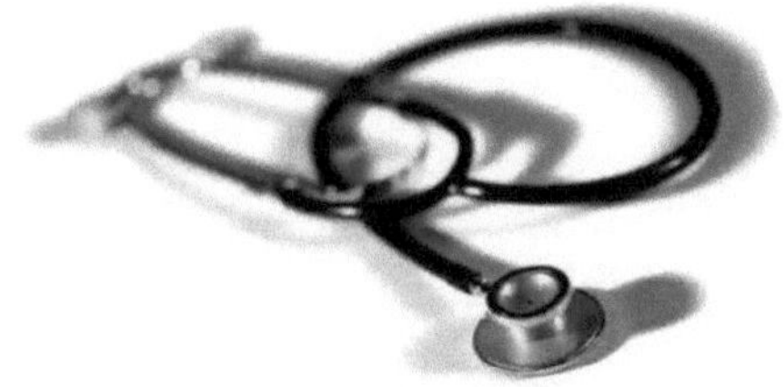

DEDICATION.

To my husband and daughters for pushing me day after day to continue moving forward.

To my fathers for always accompanying me.

My sister and nieces for their contagious joy in every work they started.

A la DraC. Anadely Gámez Pérez for her unconditional support and for being a source of permanent inspiration in our daily work.

Al DrCs. Porfirio Hernández Ramírez, tutor of this work, for motivating us to Investigate in the new world of regenerative medicine in Cuba.

Al Lic. Francisco González Cordero and the MCs. Lic. Elena López González for her dedication to collaborating in the realization of this work.

THANKS

Thank you to my colleagues whose trust and loyalty made this investigation possible. I'm struggling especially with the patients, who always taught me a lot when I heard them.

I owe special gratitude to all the staff at the Blood Bank of the Comandante Pinares Hospital who form part of the Regenerative Medicine team who, with intelligence and volun- tary, make it possible to achieve the results we show today in several investigative lines.

Thanks.

SUMMARY

Wheel osteoarthritis (OAR) is the most frequent cause of arthritis in the population over 55 years of age. In order to evaluate the effectiveness of allogeneic platelet lysate in OAR, a quasi-experimental study with simultaneous control was carried out at the General Teaching Hospital **"Comandante Pinares", in the period** 2009 to 2016. The sample consisted of 485 patients, 272 treated with allogeneic platelet lysate (studio), 213 conventionally treated (control). Women over 50 years old predominated. The most frequent comorbidities, arterial hypertension, diabetes mellitus, epilcpsy, did not make it impossible to perform the implant due to the use of allogeneic lysate. instability in the wheel, quadriceps hypotrophy. The intensity of pain decreased in 220 patients six months after the implant, gait improved, the patient's integral response following clinical and imaging recovery was good in the study group, recovery of joint space was evident with improvement of the joint surfaces and the bone density, the subchondral cysts disappeared. The allogeneic platelet lysate was effective and efficient in achieving the reincorporation of patients into their usual work activities.

TABLE OF CONTENT

INTRODUCTION

Rod osteoarthritis (RAO) is also known as gonarthrosis and is a non-inflammatory degenerative joint disease that is characterized by degeneration of the articular cartilage, subchondral sclerosis, formation of osteophytes and alteration of soft parts such as: synovial membrane, joint capsule, ligaments y muscles (1,2).

The increase in life expectancy and the greater physical demand that affects the affected population means that currently the disease is observed with greater frequency and intensity (3,4).

The United Nations Organization (UN) reports an increase in life expectancy, in 1950 there were around 200 million people aged 60 or older, which increased in 1975 to 350 million, in the year 2000 this increased to 590 million and for By 2025 there will be 1,100 million people in this age group. It is estimated that mayors aged 60 by 2025 will represent approximately 13.7% of the world population (5.6).

According to data from the National Statistics Office in Cuba in 2015, 2,158,703 people were 60 years old; of them: 85,461 belonging to the province of Artemisa, which is located in the third largest population of inhabitants of the third city per square kilometer. On the other hand, people between 40 and 59 years old in 2015, spent 3,566,081 in the country, and in the province of Artemisa 158,068.

The OAR generally affects patients for over 40 years and a large number of people are exposed to suffering from their symptoms and signs (7).

The World Health Organization (WHO) estimates that this disease affects at least 10% of the population over 60 years, and more than 20 million inhabitants in the Americas (6-8).

It was not until the 1980s that in Spain Dr Anitua and collaborators began to deepen the study of platelets as a therapeutic alternative in the approach to this condition (9).

From the year 2004, with the introduction of regenerative medicine in Cuba, a stage of scientific development began linked to the generation of regenerative processes capable of focusing on possible solutions for those diseases with rapid evolution. Investigations carried out in Cuba showed that the prevalence of OAR was 20.4% in a studied population (10).

Platelets have been used in several investigations with impactful results and especially in orthopedics, some researchers consider that an adequate supply of circulating platelets is essential to maintain vascular integrity and facilitate their regenerative capacity. The normal range of platelet count in humans is 150 $x10^{9}$ /L to 400 $x10^{9}$ /L. Its function in hemostasis is indisputable and is a natural source of CF (11,12).

The growth factors and cytokines that come from platelet granules perform an important function within this chain of regenerative events. Currently, 62 families of a wide variety of polypeptides are known to perform functions to control processes that must lead to cartilage regeneration (12-14).

The possibility of counting on the knowledge of the ultrastructural elements visualized in the platelets has allowed us to correlate them with some of their functions and to progressively discover the platelet secretome (9).

Several studies demonstrate the usefulness of platelets in orthopedics, aesthetic surgery and postphlebitic ulcers (15,16).

The behavior of the OAR, in terms of incidence, gender predominance and age with greater frequency of appearance, is similar in different countries, as well as the cost that represents the treatment.

The implant on the wheel began at the Hospital General Comandante Pinares in 2009, by specialists trained at the Hospital Nacional Enrique Cabrera and at the IHI. Later, this treatment method was extended to the rest of hospitals in Cuba (10).

This investigation forms part of the project associated with the program of the Hospital Comandante Pinares de San Cristóbal, Artemisa. This allowed us to establish action guidelines at the different levels of care of the Cuban health system in order to favor patients with RAO, in addition to Artemisa being one of the provinces with the highest population aging, which is why an increasing trend is to be expected of the illness . The previous one leads to the definition of the research problem and working hypotheses.

Planting the Problem

The investigation proposes the purpose of answering the following question: ^How effective is the allogeneic platelet lysate implant in patients with osteoarthritis of the rod?

It constitutes a fundamental element of this work to evaluate the effective results of its use in terms of an adequate regeneration of the joint cartilage with a greater exploitation of the potentialities that the platelet lysate offers, once knowing its main characteristics and peculiarities.

I- HYPOTHESIS

By implanting the allogeneic platelet lysate in patients with osteoarthritis of the rod, the regeneration of the articular cartilage will be accelerated through the supply of multiple platelet growth factors that stimulate platelet repair.

II- GOALS

GENERAL

> Evaluate the effectiveness of allogeneic platelet lysate in the treatment of **wheel osteoarthritis at the "Comandante Pinares" General Teaching Hospital of San Cristóbal, Artemisa (2009-2016).**

SPECIFIC

1. Characterize some clinical and epidemiological variables in patients with osteoarthritis.
2. Describe the comorbidities associated in patients with osteoarthritis of the rod.
3. Compare the evolution of symptoms and signs before and after the implant as well as the clinical and radiological response to treatment.
4. Identify adverse effects generated by the treatment.
5. Evaluate the function of the wheel using the WOMAC scale, before and after the implant with allogeneic platelets.
6. Determine the cost of infiltration with allogeneic platelet lysate in relation to conventional treatment of osteoarthritis.

Main contributions of the thesis

The work provides elements that allow us to deepen the knowledge of the usefulness of platelet lysate in the treatment of osteoarthrosis of the rod, due to the absence of similar investigations in the country and few communications in the international literature.

Scientific news

In this work, the usefulness of allogeneic platelet lysate in patients with osteoarthrosis of the rod was **established for the first time in Cuba .** The use of this blood component represents a greater burden in outpatient treatment, as this condition constitutes a health problem primarily in third-age patients.

This is a novel investigation with great impact in the field of medicine in general. Many of these patients have disability, their evolution is rapid and they have a very high risk of complications. According to what is mentioned in the literature consulted, there is no treatment that restores functionality quickly and effectively.

Patients receive conventional medical-surgical treatment and in accordance with international statistics and it is necessary to act in the earliest stages of the illness.

From where we know, therapy with platelets or platelet components in osteoarthritis of the rod has been carried out in Spain, Argentina, Colombia and more recently in Cuba, with encouraging results from the clinical point of view and with very few adverse effects.

The usefulness of allogeneic platelet lysate therapy in this type of patients represents a major scientific impact on the ground at national and international level.

Social value

This procedure manages to reduce the number of cases that require hospital admission and early retirement, maintaining their physical independence, which has a significant impact on the physical state and quality of life of patients with this illness.

Economic value

The application of the method that is analyzed in this investigation contributes to a lower consumption of medicines and avoids expenses for surgical treatment in cases that require conventional treatment. Furthermore, in the case of the group that uses depreciated platelets, which have lost their hemostatic function, these constitute low levels in blood banks and taking advantage of the regenerative potential of this product, it is considered as recovered raw material. Therefore, its recovery as a result represents what in the economic aspect could be considered as a **waste of raw materials** .

Practical value

The platelet lysate obtained from allogeneic platelets is a safe, accessible and beneficial element in the treatment of osteoarthritis of the rod, it constitutes a major tool that, in addition to specific treatment in accordance with the etiology of the disease, contributes to accelerating the regeneration of the articular cartilage .

CHAPTER 1

THEORETICAL FRAMEWORK

Currently, the treatment of patients with wheel osteoarthritis with allogeneic platelet lysate has aroused interest due to the great expectation that has been raised regarding its effectiveness. For this reason, different aspects related to the disease are addressed in a detailed and updated way, which facilitates the understanding and interpretation of the investigation.

1.1 Rodilla osteoarthritis. Definition. Classification

Rod osteoarthritis (RAO), popularly known as «joint wear», is a common disease of middle age, constituting one of the main causes of disability. The development of the illness is slow and the pain progresses over time. Although there is no cure, there are several treatment options that help control the pain, restore the functionality of the wheel and lead a satisfactory life (17).

The simplest classification is based on etiology, which divides them into primary

and secondary, the latter as a result of previous traumas, infections, surgeries, among others (18,19).

There is little interrelationship in some patients between symptoms and signs, radiographic and arthroscopic hallmarks and it is very difficult to carry out a classification that adjusts to these elements. The radiographic classifications of the OAR are inaccurate, especially in the first stages (20).

The use of arthroscopy allows for a more detailed description of the magnitude and extent of the lesion, as well as the early detection of reblading and fibrillation. Reason why most researchers prefer arthroscopic classifications. The Outerbridge RE classification is the most used from a practical point of view according to the Alomban AS (17,19) in addition to being a classification compatible with others widely used worldwide. In this investigation we used Kellgren and Lawrence.

1.1.2 . Physiopathology

The wear of the cartilage and, therefore, the origin of the disease is produced by a sum of mechanical and biochemical factors (20).

Firstly, overload of pressure on a cartilage, or normal force on an altered cartilage can cause cracks on the surface of the cartilage and subsequently a progressive loss of the tissue.

Secondly, these mechanical forces can provide the presence of some proteins that, finally, are responsible for the destruction of different components of the cartilage (collagen and proteoglycans) and the progression of the disease (21).

It is accepted that in the normal cartilage, there is a balance between the synthesis and degradation of the matrix molecules. In pathological conditions, such as arthrosis, the dominant process is catabolism, with progressive and irreversible destruction of the cartilage. The first evidence of degradation is the fibrillation of the articular surface and the loss of glycoproteins (22).

Damage to the collagen structure causes the water content (edema) of the tissue to increase. In later stages, the fibrillation process causes fissures and ruptures in the cartilage that can extend to the subchondral hue.

In patients with long evolution, pathological changes are associated in the tissues of the joint such as subchondral cysts, osteophytes and the replacement of hyaline cartilage by fibrocartilage.

The cartilage of patients with arthrosis from the histological point of view is heterogeneous, with areas of cellular proliferation and high synthetic activity (indicative of reparative activity), with areas of degradation, necrosis and inflammation (23).

Furthermore, high levels of proteinases (enzymes) that degrade the matrix have been detected, known as: metalloproteinases (MMP), of which in particular are stromelysin (MMP3) and collagenase (MMP1), which are capable of degrading glucosaminoglycans, collagen and other matrix proteins. The presence in the synovial fluid of fragments of the extracellular matrix, proteolytic enzymes and cytokines represent biological markers of the disease (24).

Biomechanical changes in the diseased tissue cause a significant reduction in the elastic property of the cartilage. On the other hand, the high water content makes the fabric more compressible and permeable. Although the superficial layers play an important role in supporting loads in the healthy and intact cartilage, the fibrillation in the superficial zone generates tensions and greater deformities in the solid matrix and a decrease in the capacity to support weight loads (25) .

1.1.3 Diagnosis

It has been decided that the Spanish Society of Rheumatology (SER) has issued the criterion that the diagnosis of the disease is carried out through a clinical interview (26).

There are some tests that help the specialist complete the study. Using an x-ray, the doctor can distinguish the osteophytes, the pressure of the cartilage, the subchondral geodes and the asymmetrical diminution of the joint space, clear symptoms of RAO.

Other tests that can be used in exceptional cases are CT and magnetic resonance imaging when the doctor has doubts about the origin of the process or is studying in a complementary way other problems, such as disc extrusion in a spondyloarthrosis or a meniscal tear in an OAR.

Finally, high-resolution ultrasound has been incorporated as a very effective diagnostic tool because it reveals the soft parts surrounding the joint, as well as whether there is inflammation or injury in some of them and distinguishing whether the profile of the bone is changing(26 ,27).

1.1.4 Clinical manifestations of illness

Clinically, this condition is characterized by joint pain, stiffness, limited movement, and varying degrees of inflammation (28). On the other hand, it is also characterized by an imbalance between anabolic and catabolic processes (27), which results in progressive damage to the cartilage, and ultimately the patient's disability.

1.1.5 Conservative Therapy

Conservative treatment in the management of wheel osteoarthritis constitutes a fundamental variety, especially in outpatient management in the areas of primary and secondary health. An updated bibliographic review was carried out on forms of treatment consisting of: lifestyle modification, rehabilitation, use of footwear, orthosis, support devices,

analgesics, anti-inflammatory drugs, intraarticular steroids and viscosupplementation (29).

1.1.5.1 Lifestyle modification

Patient education is vitally important for lifestyle modification to be effective. You should avoid all activities with a high demand for energy and ensure adequate rest to alleviate symptoms. Obesity is a risk factor for osteoarthritis and its symptoms, exercise that involves running or jumping should be avoided; However, low-impact exercises like swimming and cycling constitute suitable variants. The reduction in exercise when climbing and lowering stairs significantly reduces the pain of patellofemoral osteoarthritis (27,30).

1.1.5.2 Rehabilitation

The need to prescribe rehabilitation therapy to the patient depends on the degree and severity of the illness as well as the patient's expectations. Exercises are recommended to maintain the range of movement of the joint and in this way contractures are prevented or reduced.

The rehabilitation method can be combined with the application of heat, hydrotherapy, ultrasound and cryotherapy. The duration and frequency must be adjusted for each patient (31).

1.1.5.3 Footwear

The use of shoes and other devices can reduce compression forces at the level of the wheel joint. Reducing the weight load in the affected compartment considerably reduces the pain.

Other studies show that between 75 and 85% of patients with osteoarthritis of the medial compartment, treated by elevating the sole of the shoe, showed significant improvement from a statistical point of view. The shoe must be placed on the opposite side of the injury to avoid reducing the compression strength of the affected compartment. In the case of patellofemoral osteoarthritis, low-heeled and high-sole shoes can be used (31,32).

1.1.5.4 Orthosis

Even though the use of orthosis does not alter the alignment of the rod forces, this treatment method provides a sensation of stability to the patient. These external application devices comply with the principle of three points of support: a force applied at the center of the wheel and the other two, opposing forces in a proximal and distal direction to the wheel. In case of varus deformity, the device must be placed in valgus to reduce the forces on the medial side.

Some authors claim that 50% of patients show improvement after applying and using the orthosis for 7 hours a day and 5 days a week (33). This method has the inconvenience of being expensive ($800-1,000) and some patients refuse to use it during the day. However, it is a very reasonable alternative for young patients or for those who refuse osteotomy and rod arthroplasty (33,34).

1.1.5.5 Support devices

The use of a crutch or stick on the contralateral side is an effective method for reducing strength and symptoms caused by wheel osteoarthritis. This method is very effective in the acute phase in patients with antalgic gait, caused by pain and inflammation at times (9,16). However, it is not fully accepted by patients because many opine on the loss of independence (34).

1.1.5.1 Pharmacological treatment

Pharmacological modality includes the use of analgesics, non-steroidal anti-inflammatory agents, chondroprotective agents or supplements, intraarticular injection of steroids and viscosupplementation (34,35).

1.1.5.2 Painkillers

Although the relationship between pain and osteoarthritis is poor, there is no doubt that relief is the most important element in therapy. Due to the presence of few undesirable effects and its effectiveness, paracetamol is the analgesic of choice for orthopedics and rheumatologists. The recommended dose is 650 mg every 6 hours with a maximum dose of 4,000 mg per day (34,36).

1.1.5.3 "Non-steroidal" anti-inflammatory drugs

The mechanism of action of all "non-steroidal" anti-inflammatory drugs (NSAIDs) consists of interrupting the synthesis of prostaglandins through the inhibition of the cyclooxygenase enzyme (COX). In the 90s, 2 forms of COX were identified (COX-1 and COX-2). COX-1 is present in the stomach and kidneys of healthy people through the production of prostaglandins. The COX-2 enzyme is induced in the joints of patients with inflammatory arthritis, through the production of prostaglandins, which can cause or worsen inflammation. In theory, NSAIDs that have selective inhibition of COX-2 without inhibition of COX-1 should have anti-inflammatory activity without gastrointestinal or toxic renal effects (37).

NSAIDs have three major pharmacological actions: anti-inflammatory, analgesic-antipyretic and also behave as an antiplatelet agent (37).

- Anti-inflammatory action: a decrease in vasodilatory prostaglandins PGE2, PGI2 is produced, which often decreases vasodilation and edema.
- Analgesic-antipyretic effect: the decrease in proteoglycans causes less sensation in the nerve endings of inflammatory mediators, generating additional temperature regulatory mechanisms.
- Antiplatelet effect: this is short, if it is planned that 24 hours after suspension, the bleeding time returns to normal, not with aspirin whose action can last from 10 to 12 days. All NSAIDs are eliminated by hepatic biotransformation and are excreted through the kidney (37,38).

Among the undesirable effects are: dyspepsia, which is the most frequent of all, gastrointestinal ulcers, nephrotoxicity and hepatotoxicity as well as cardiac failure. They are generally related to high doses and advanced age (39).

Based on the above, NSAIDs are contraindicated in gastrointestinal, hepatic and renal diseases and in patients undergoing anticoagulation treatment.

1.1.5.9 Chondroprotective agents

Glucosamine and chondroitin sulfate are endogenous molecules of the articular cartilage with synergistic action when administered together. Glucosamine stimulates the metabolism of the chondrocyte and synodite, in addition, it inhibits degrading enzymes and prevents the formation of fibrin thrombi in periarticular tissues. Approximately 87% of the administered dose of glucosamine is absorbed at the intestinal level and is excreted via the kidneys (40,41).

Chondroitin sulfate is important to promote the union of collagen fibers. Its protective effect is caused by the inhibition of degrading enzymes that cause rupture of the articular cartilage. Furthermore, chondrite sulfate is an effective inhibitor of thrombus formation, which affects periarticular tissues and reduces blood supply to the synovial and subchondral bones (42).

The recommended dosage is 1 g of glucosamine and 1,200 mg of chondroitin sulfate per day (43).

1.1.5.10 Use of intraarticular steroids

Intraarticular injection of steroids is of great help in patients who have primarily failed to use analgesics and anti-inflammatory drugs or in those who are contraindicated.

They are indicated for persistent inflammation and the presence of pain in patients with osteoarthritis who do not respond to other treatment modalities within a period of 6 to 8 weeks (43-45).

Intraarticular steroids are potent anti-inflammatory drugs with minimal risk of systemic effects or complications. There are 2 types of preparations: microcrystalline and crystalline. Among the microcrystalline substances are: triamcinolone, methylprednisolone and hydrocortisone acetate which have the advantage of having a slower absorption and a longer effect in comparison with crystalline substances such as betamethasone (46).

Previous joint aspiration is not recommended unless the patient has joint inflammation. Using this modality can provide pain relief for up to 6 months or more. On occasion, intraarticular injections should not be more than 3 or 4 per year because after this dose they begin to diminish their effect (46,47).

The main complications with the reference method include atrophy of subcutaneous fat and changes in skin pigmentation. The most important contraindications are: recent fractures or microtraumas as well as signs of a local infectious process (47).

1.1.5.11 Viscosupplementation

The injection of hyaluronate or viscosupplementation, called as it favors the viscoelasticity of synovial fluid, is another variety of treatment available for osteoarthritis of the rod . There are currently 2 agents

Hyalgan and Synvisc available. Three to five weekly injections are generally used. These agents promote viscoelasticity, the synovial tissue is more effective in absorbing weight loads and lubricating the joint surfaces. Other effects of viscosupplementation include the synthesis of hyaluronate acid by type A cells, the synthesis of proteoglycans by chondrocytes, anti-inflammatory and analgesic effects (48). Depending on the severity of the OAR, pain relief may last up to 6 months. After administration, the patient must avoid weight bearing for 48 hours (49).

The normal amount of synovial fluid in the joint is 2 mL with a concentration of hyaluronic acid that varies from 2.5 to 4 mg per mL. In patients with osteoarthritis of the rod, the concentration of hyaluronic acid is reduced to less than a third of the normal amount. Furthermore, the molecular size of hyaluronic acid is reduced and the interaction between the molecules of this acid is reduced. These changes cause modifications in the elastic properties of the synovial fluid and in this way, the loss of lubrication originates greater stress in the strengths of friction with ruptures of the collagen fibers that are essential for the integration of the articular cartilage (50,51).

1.2 State of musculoskeletal diseases in Latin America.

The World Health Organization considers the decade from 2010 to 2020 as the Hueso and Articulación. They are here to highlight the importance of musculoskeletal illnesses. Four diseases are considered to be of special relevance: a) rheumatoid arthritis, b) osteoporosis, c) osteoarthritis and d) pain in the lower part of the back (52). The impact of this decade will have to be critically assessed in different regions of the world. In Latin America it does not seem to have been especially successful, its first five years in study.

Information from several studies in Latin America highlights several relevant data that undoubtedly emphasize the importance of these illnesses. The prevalence of musculoskeletal pain is present in approximately 25% of individuals surveyed at the community level. Many of these patients are not served by the health systems. Patients who resort to medical care are often attended by a general doctor, who usually prescribes non-steroidal anti-inflammatory drugs. Several illnesses that should be managed by a rheumatologist are not diagnosed. The delay in the remission to specialists of illnesses such as rheumatoid arthritis has been cataloged as a date of poor prognosis. Spain has had successful educational experiments for general physicians to improve diagnostic quality and timely referral of patients to specialized treatment. A reduction has also been shown in the time to start the first disease-modifying antirheumatic drug in rheumatoid arthritis. Similar examples should be promoted in Latin America and are part of an agenda with recommendations issued by the GLADAR and PANLAR group (53,54).

The costs and complexity of regional museums must be considered and the benefits of information that can be used to support regional needs must be evaluated (55) . The impact of this information on health policies is likely to be reflected after several years of coordinated and intense work.

Future trends call on us to pay attention to the urgent need to take the aging of the population seriously. Leading authors in the area of aging have pointed out that this phenomenon has special characteristics in Latin America and the Caribbean, namely: a) the speed of aging will be especially fast in this region. If you think that in the year 2030, the population older than 60 years will be 2.5 to 3.5 times larger when compared to the figures from the year 2000; b) this region has a dislocation between aging and adequate standards of life. If it is compared with other populations, such as the European, Latin American and Caribbean populations, they will reach adulthood without having enjoyed the life standards of other populations and it is postulated that they could be associated with less favorable aging; c) the sociopolitical context and institutional volatility significantly compromise the most optimistic predictions. It is thought that we do not have until now adequate preparation to face the challenges that population aging imposes on our region (55-58).

1.3 Current epidemiological status of osteoarthritis in Cuba

In Cuba, the first epidemiological studies addressing the prevalence of rheumatic diseases in the community found that osteoarthritis was the most common, at 20.41%. It also evaluated associated disability and in the case of osteoarthritis it was strongly associated with some degree of disability (57).

In our country, the morbidity of this disease is not sufficiently studied, nor is the disability associated with it. Even considering the aging process, seen as an increase in the proportion of people aged 60 and more in relation to the total population, it has been developing and deepening in recent years.

Cuba has gone from 11.3 percent of people aged 60 and older in 1985 to 17.0 percent in 2008, which indicates its location in Group III of aging (more than 15.0% of the population of 60 years and more in total). Therefore, in 23 years, aging has increased by 5.7 percentage points

Among the most aged municipalities in the country are Plaza de la Revolución, Diez de Octubre and Placetas, with 25.4, 22.8 and 22.8%, Artemisa today occupies third place in population aging of Adult Mayors, respectively. The three territories present indicators V/J (relationship between the number of people aged 60 and over (V) and the number of children and young people aged 0 to 14, (J) (per 1000)) and V/A (relationship between the number of people aged 60 and more and adults between

15 and 59 years old, (A) (per 1000) less favorable people across the country, and the highest rates of aging (7).

The municipality of Artemisa, due to its population aging, presents a high morbidity due to OAR, considering these aspects and knowing the regenerative potential of platelets, finding a hopeful solution for this invalidating disease in the results of this investigation.

1.4 The plaques, their discovery and functions

The platelets were the last to be discovered of the 3 major elements of blood, their identification was attributed to the French doctor Alfred Donne, in 1842. It was the German anatomist Max Schultze who confirmed the existence of these elements and was the first to make them description. Years later, George Hayem in 1878 and Giulio Bizzorero in 1882, provided more **information. Bizzorero called "piastrine", small plates, these new corpuscles, which were later called "plaquettes" in French, "platelets" in English and consequently, platelets in Spanish (59).**

Platelets were described as **"spherules" smaller than** hematites, which on occasions appeared as aggregates and could participate in the formation of a fibrous material; Furthermore, it was demonstrated that these structures were anucleate. The continuation of his studies managed to provide valuable information on platelet intervention in the blood coagulation process (60).
The application of optical microscopy facilitates the study of the shape of platelets, but the greatest advances were obtained in time after the introduction of electronic microscopy and transmission that allowed a better characterization of the platelet structure (61,62).

1.5 Platelets as a source of growth factors

Platelets are viable fragments that are incorporated into each traumatic or surgical wound.
According to its characteristics and therapeutic possibilities, it has been used for different purposes.
In the United States, the use of platelet blood components originating in Blood Banks (Red Cross) was reported and in Europe, thrombin of bovine origin was used before relating it to the prions with Creunfeld_Jakob disease (63-66).

Since understanding the function of platelets, work has been carried out on their use in the development of tissue regeneration. The clinical use of CP, platelet-rich plasma (PRP) and platelet lysate (LP) has shown double the speed of bone formation and has increased the density of bone injections by 20%.

Platelets contain multiple CFs, including: PDGF, PDGF- β , IGF, EGF, as well as other factors that include epidermal growth factor (EGF) and hepatocyte growth factor (HGF).

Radiologically and histologically it has been shown that the use of PRP concentrate can be used to accelerate osteointegration in titanium implants (67).

The pharmaceutical industry promoted the development of products based on PDGF, being approved in 1997. It is necessary to consider that when using the so-called platelet patch, the platelet clot, in soil high concentrations of PDGF are applied as well as TGF β and VEGF, which can increase adhesion and enhance its effect (67,68).

However, the platelet lysate in soil contains small amounts of platelets and other FC, but also plasma with fibrin that influences healing. Fibrin acts as a provisional scaffold for cellular migration and differentiation of mother cells and also functions as biological attachment (69).

As previously mentioned, the LP is frequently used today for the healing of defects, bone consolidation and osteointegration (70).

The natural and immediate response of the organism to damaged tissue is the accumulation of a large number of activated platelets at the injured site. Activated platelets interact at various levels within the coagulation cascade, and a clot quickly forms.

The granules contained in platelets release FC and cytokines. These proteins, which include PDGF, TGF, VEGF and EGF, attract macrophages, mesenchymal cells, osteoblasts and cells responsible for removing necrotic tissue. The released proteins act as chemotactic, morphogenetic and mitogenic agents. The secretion of presynthesized proteins occurs within the first 10 minutes of platelet activation, and more than 95% are secreted within the first hour. Platelets continue to secrete these proteins for an average of five to 10 days and up to 21 days after being extracted by donation. Because a supraphysiological dose of activated platelets can theoretically accelerate the healing process, thus inhibiting bacterial growth (65).

It is a technological possibility to take a volume of venous blood of 60 mL from the patient and process PRP as another alternative.

The use of different biological elements that contribute to CF, whether they are of natural origin or as a result of genetic recombination, has modified the treatment of chronic lesions, both in orthopedic surgery and in maxillofacial surgery and in the range of postphlebitic ulcerative lesions (14). The usefulness of these plates in other specialties, as already mentioned, constitutes a proven fact today.

The use of PRP has beneficial effects in joint surgeries that require filling a bone defect at the time of performing an arthroplasty or in the case of complicated fractures that fail to consolidate (71,72).

It is important to remember the principles of basic surgery, such as biomechanical stability, tissue coverage, conservation of vascularization, eradication of infection, an ideal environment for the repair of bones and ulcers. The possibility of carrying out the treatment in a clinic, office or patient's home allows for a wider range of uses.

1.6 Biological activity of the main platelet growth factors

The first reference to the existence of bioactive substances, characterized as growth factors, was called (EGF) and was carried out by the same group of scientists who discovered the so-called nerve tissue growth factor, (NGF) (73,74).

These substances have the ability to stimulate mitosis, proliferation (scarring) and angiogenesis, and promote chemotactism, among other properties (75).

The so-called cellular communication is the result of the investigation of these factors, which constitutes an advance in the understanding of this process (74).

The first to demonstrate the beneficial effects of the so-called Platelet Derived Growth Factor,

(PDGF) in the treatment of chronic herides, was Knighton's work carried out on the basis of a randomized study (75).

In table 1, the effect, biological action or both properties of each FC are summarized in a summarized way, which can in advance justify the reason for scarring and the reproduction capacity of the stages of coagulation, of these factors.

Table 1. Activity of bioactive molecules

Bioactive molecule	Biological activity
Growth factor derived from las platelets (FCDP)	- Potent mitogen for fibroblasts, arterial smooth muscle cells, chondrocytes, epithelial and endothelial cells - Potent chemotactic effect for hematopoietic and mesenchymal cells, - Stimulates chemotaxis and activation of muscle macrophages and fibroblasts - Activates transforming growth factor b to stimulate macrophages and neutrophils - Type 1 collagen synthesis - Angiogenesis (indirectly)
Growth factor vascular endothelial (FCEV)	- Stimulates proliferation of macrovascular endothelial cells - Potent angiogenic - Induce synthesis of metalloproteins that degrade interstitial collagen
Transforming growth factor beta **(FCT β)**	- Stimulates fibroblastic chemotaxis, proliferation and collagen synthesis - Inhibits the formation of osteoclasts and bone reabsorption - Reduction of dermal scarring - Inhibits the growth of fibroblasts, epithelial cells,

	endothelial cells, neuronal cells, some types of hematopoietic cells and keratinocytes
	- Antagonist of the biological activity of the FCE, he FCDPyel FCFa - Promotes angiogenesis
Growth factor similar to insulin types I and II (FCI-I and FCI-II)	- Fibroblast growth - Cell mitogenesis and differentiation mesenchymal and coating - Mitogenic *in vitro* for some mesodermal cells - Promotes collagen and prostaglandin E2 synthesis in fibroblasts - Stimulates collagen and matrix synthesis by bone cells, regulating the metabolism of the articular cartilage.
Acidic and basic fibroblast growth factor (FCFa and FCFb)	*FCFa:* participates in the proliferation and differentiation of osteoblasts and inhibition of osteoblasts - Promotes angiogenesis and cell migration - Mitogen for skin-derived keratinocytes, dermal fibroblasts and vascular endothelial cells FCFb: stimulates the growth of fibroblasts, myoblasts, osteoblasts, neuronal cells, endothelial cells, keratinocytes and chondrocytes - Increases fibronectin production - Stimulates angiogenesis, cell proliferation
	endothelial cells and collagen synthesis - Matrix synthesis. Epithelialization and production of FC of keratinocytes and retraction of herides

Growth factor epidermal (FCE)	- Mitogenic function (proliferation, differentiation and migration) of epidermal cells, epithelial cells, fibroblasts, embryonic cells. In addition, nasal cells, glia from mesenchymal cells - Chemotactics of fibroblasts and epithelial cells - Stimulates re-epithelization - Increases angiogenesis - Influences the synthesis and renewal of the extracellular matrix - Proapoptotic

Fuente: Tomada de Fernández Delgado N, et al. 2012

1.7 Cuba is a particular scenario, which offers safe allogeneic blood platelet growth factors

There are basic elements to conceptualize a blood bank. Among them are the discovery of blood groups, as well as the development of anticoagulant solutions necessary for blood collection, the perfection of blood infusion equipment such as plastic bags with anticoagulants and disposable equipment that allows it preserve the blood for several weeks in refrigeration. It is an institution where blood is collected, blood components are produced, in addition to regulating and ensuring the transfusion of the same to patients who need it (76).

The ethical principles have always been present in the collection, the process and the transfusion of blood and its components. Fundamentally oriented towards the protection of the donor and recipient of blood.

The International Society for Blood Transfusion developed the Code of Ethics for the donation and transfusion of blood in 1980, which was approved by the XXIV International Conference of La Cruz Roja in 1989. Voluntary blood donation is not a simple idealistic thing , is a primordial ethical question. For this reason, the ethical principles of voluntariness, anonymity and altruism of blood donors were ratified by consensus (77). The performance of the activity of the Blood Banks requires vitally for the success of the correct and timely application of the principles of bioethics.

The donation of blood is an act in which the principle of beneficence has a dual purpose: not to cause harm to the donor or the recipient of the blood. In this way, in the interrogation, physical examination and laboratory studies that are carried out by the donor, we seek to detect antecedents, symptoms, signs or laboratory parameters that could damage any of them.

The method of self-exclusion of the donor, after receiving written information on some of the possible causes that could invalidate him as a donor (belonging to risky groups such as drug addicts, promiscuous people, etc.), he can decline the act of donating or sending The newsletter that your blood is risky. This way, the donor avoids having to answer embarrassing questions (78).

The written informed consent is the document where the donor of the security and veracity of the donation he performs at that moment, also authorizes the use of his blood after it is verified that its use is safe, and is used more frequently.

Secondly, the remunerated donation can cause risks for the donor, because due to economic interests it can hide pathological situations that can damage the state of health in the donor's condition, the donation more frequently than the admitted one, and violating the recommended time periods between one or another donation. On the other hand, donors must receive compensation, in the event of an accident or complication associated with donating blood.

In Cuba there are blood banks, provincial and municipal, in accordance with the assistance needs, the National Group of Hematology and Blood Banks was created that directs the training of specialist doctors, other professionals dedicated to the activity and average technicians of this specialty. The National Blood of Cuba Program summarizes all the aspirations of this field. On the other hand, the State Center for Medication Control of the Ministry of Public Health dictates regulations that ensure the protection of donors and recipients in accordance with the ethical principles of donation and blood transfusion (78).

The creation of research centers at the scientific center has allowed the development of innovative detection systems for hepatitis B and C viruses, and the achievement of soon introducing new studies to determine the presence of other viruses, in addition to the Human Immunodeficiency virus , HIV, with those who research all blood donations from the country.

These tests ensure the safety of blood products in recipients, as well as allowing the health of the Cuban population of blood donors to be monitored (76).

Voluntary and unpaid donation has characterized blood donation in Cuba. Thanks to this achievement, the country is satisfied with blood products to support humanitarian projects such as transplantation, cardiovascular surgery, oncology and others. This is due to the universal and free nature of the health system and the education achieved in Cuba, as well as the active participation of mass organizations and the entire community in this task.

The implementation in Cuban blood banks of virus detection techniques guarantees safe blood supply to patients, in accordance with the Alliance for Hematological Security (79).

The use of treatment with allogeneic platelets, as a source of lysate is common in other countries, obtaining from autologous platelets even with incomparable safety, is considered, as an inconvenience of this method of treatment, the need to extract a minimum of 400 ml of blood to the patient in order to obtain a volume of platelet concentrate sufficient for the preparation of cylinders of pentacalcium phosphate agglutinated with fibrin. This requirement limits the indications for this treatment in small children, in which the extraction of this volume of blood would be logically conditioned to the total blood volume of the patient, in addition to those who need higher and frequent doses, as is the case of the sick. with ulcerative lesions (80).

1.8 Other clinical applications of platelets or platelet growth factors

The use of platelets has extended into different fields of medicine. These extrahemostatic actions have led to rapid solutions to phenomena whose duration lasts for a long time (81-83).

Several authors considered its indication in the specialty of orthopedics with favorable results (84-87) among them:

- Osteoarthritis
- Bone defects
- Tendinitis and peritendinitis
- Pseudoarthrosis
- Meniscus rupture
- Plantar fasciitis
- Bone insertions
- Epicondylitis
- Ligament injuries
- Muscle injuries

- Arthrodesis of vertebral bodies

- Delay in consolidation fractures.

Encouraging results have been described in Stomatology and Maxillofacial Surgery (88-93). Which relate to the continuation:

Periodontal defects (gingival retraction and others)

Endodontics

Alveolar regeneration

dentoalveolar surgery

As a tissue adhesive

Implantology

Buconasales communications

Replenishment of bone defects

Prevention of dry alveolitis after third molar extraction.

Dermatology has been useful in its use in different entities (94,95).

For example:

Epithelial healing

Chronic ulcers

Pressure ulcers.

Bedsores, androgenic alopecia.

Angiology has been one of the specialties most benefited from the use of platelets, in the entities that are most noted below, several authors have established criteria for its effectiveness (12, 96, 97).

Diabetic pie

Vascular ulcers

Peripheral arterial insufficiency

Several articles also relate the benefits that the use of platelets or their components in aesthetic surgery brings, with indications that will be further detailed (1, 61,98).

- Facial tissue lifting
- Rhytidectomies
- Blepharoplasties
- Facial rejuvenation
- Breast reconstruction

In Oftalmología good results are described in (99).

- Corneal injuries
- Severe dry eye
- Ocular surface dysfunction syndrome after refractive surgery
- LASIK (Laser-Assisted in Situ Keratomileusis)
- Eye burns
- Bacterial keratoconjunctivitis
- Recurrent keratitis.
- Sjogren's syndrome
- Severe ophthalmic injury injection after bone marrow transplant.

Other reports coincide with the report regarding the effectiveness of the use of this bioactive substance in ocular diseases (44, 82,100).

Sports medicine has also incorporated the use of platelets as an efficient alternative for the rapid recovery of athletes. With some of the lesions that lower they are related (11.87).

- Tendon and ligament injuries
- Muscle injuries due to overuse
- Joint injuries.

Other indications that satisfactory results have been obtained, expressed in international literature, have been reported by several researchers, among which it is possible to relate (101-105).

- Heirloom scarring
- Loss of soft tissue due to trauma
- Breast tissue regeneration after surgery
- Biological tissue adhesive
- Burns
- Thoracic wall closure in cardiovascular surgery

More recently, the usefulness of PRP has been demonstrated as a biological support for stromal cells extracted from the bone marrow and its possible use in cellular therapy for the regeneration of the nervous system (106-109).

1.9 Regenerative medicine in Cuba. Current therapeutic alternative

A modality employed in regenerative medicine has been, as in other countries, the use of isogroup ABO allogeneic platelets from transfusion services, which maintains current safety in pre-transfusion practice (14,110), which allows their use of platelets that haemostatically have reduced their action, but that retain their capacity to secrete growth factors and other bioactive products. This allows you to use a product until it has been developed (75).

The application of allogeneic platelets can be considered in urgent situations and when the patient has some limitation or impossibility for the extraction of blood, or when the needs that are required are greater than what an autologous donation unit provides, in quantity and frequency of use. Its fundamental drawback is the latent possibility of disease transmission, but allergic reactions are less likely to occur than could be achieved through its generally local mode of application (75). On the other hand, no significant adverse reactions have been reported with this type of application.

1.10 Clinical studies on the use of platelet lysate as a treatment for osteoarthritis and clinical evaluation scales.

The clinical studies currently available in the medical literature support the use of platelet lysate for the treatment of cartilage lesions in the rod, applying it in the form of intraarticular infiltrations. In all cases, clinical scales or indices (WOMAC, IKDC, KOOS, NRS, among others) are used to evaluate and measure the effect of treatment. According to very heterogeneous studies regarding the type of condition of treated patients, the interval of application of infiltrations, as well as the number of applications of the same, and the predominance of evaluation periods of short to medium duration (111).

CHAPTER 2

METHODOLOGICAL DISEASE

2.1 Type of studio

A quasi-experimental study was carried out with simultaneous control, in orthopedic and traumatology services together with the blood bank, of the General Teaching Hospital "Comandante Pinares", in the period between 2009 and December 2016.

2.2 Universe and exhibition

485 patients were evaluated with the diagnosis of wheel osteoarthritis with inadequate response to conventional treatment. The patients were included in 2 groups, using the simple chance method, through closed envelopes , once they offered their consent to enter the study, 272 patients received treatment with intraarticular infiltration in plates of platelet lysate obtained from negative ABO compatible allogeneic platelets for infection research tests according to officially established procedures that followed the standards for the use of blood components, but were not useful For its use as a hemostatic agent (study group), in these patients donation is contraindicated. The other 213 cases maintained conventional treatment for this condition and joined the control group.

2.3 Inclusion criteria

1. Patients aged 15 or over.
2. Patient diagnosed with rod arthrosis.
3. Patients who do not have a history of infectious processes in the affected joint within the last six months.
4. No response to conventional treatment or little benefit, without prior treatment.
5. Patients who have given informed consent to be included in the investigation.

2.4 Exclusion criteria

- Patients with illnesses that contraindicate treatment (patients with active neoplasms, neoplasms within 5 years of treatment, hepatitis B, hepatitis C, HIV infection).

- Patients with decompensated Diabetes Mellitus.
- Patients who are actively participating in other therapeutic research for this illness.
- Contraindications for local anesthesia.

2.5 Obtaining and preparing platelets and platelet lysates

Blood group determination of the ABO system was carried out on all patients to guarantee donor-recipient compatibility and production of platelet concentrate (PC) according to conventional techniques. The PRP was separated from the total blood by light centrifugation (2750 rpm x 4 to 5' at 22°C

and then rapid centrifugation (3750 rpm x 10' at 22°C) was added to obtain the CP (67).

The entire procedure from blood collection to CP preparation was carried out at a temperature of 22°C. In all cases, cooling is avoided, as it can produce platelet aggregation and reduce the performance of the preparation. The separation took place within 4 to 6 hours after phlebotomy. Enough plasma is added to the concentrate (between 50 and 70 mL) in order to maintain the pH between 6.4 and 7.4. In this way, a single unit of enteral blood must produce a concentrate with a number of platelets between 5.5×10^{10}/L and 7.5×10^{10}/L (112).

Platelet conservation in liquid phase was carried out at 4 °C for three days. After the third day, those that did not show changes in color, a platelet count was taken in the Neubauer chamber and noted in the blood bank record, then they were frozen at -30°C for an hour and subsequently thawed for six minutes in María's bathroom. This procedure was carried out three times to obtain a homogeneous lysate rich in growth factors from platelets with functional expiration and stored at -30°C. Platelets were counted again and a microbiological study was carried out on all bags, taking 1mL of the sample, after thawing quickly in a water bath, before applying the platelet lysate to the patient. Data from the bag delivered is recorded in the blood bank registry.

2.6 Treatment scheme using allogeneic platelet lysate

2.5 ml of allogeneic platelet lysate was infiltrated to the patients of the study group, into the intraarticular space via an anterolateral internal route on each roller, using a 21 gauge needle under asepsis and antisepsis conditions. The entire process was carried out on an outpatient basis. It is recommended to rest for 72 hours in cold conditions, 30 minutes 4 times a day.

2.7 Treatment scheme in the Control Group

The conventional procedure includes: It is essential to understand that up to current knowledge there is no conservative treatment of OA demonstrated to be capable of stopping or slowing down the advancement of its progression.

In relation to available pharmacological treatments, it is essential to differentiate between those that pose a finitely analgesic and those that are proposed as chondroprotectors or modulators of the disease. If paracetamol, non-steroidal anti-inflammatory drugs (NSAIDs), intraarticular corticosteroids (CIA) have been used, Glucosamine (GA) and chondroitin sulfate (CS), Hyaluronic acid.

2.8 Assessment of pain, gait and degrees of OAR

Pain was evaluated using the Visual Analogue Scale (VAS) in scheduled appointments, always by the same examiner and each patient was instructed how to carry out self-evaluation, according to the following scale:

Table 2. Scale to measure the intensity of joint pain from rollers

Scale to measure the intensity of joint pain from rollers	
0	Absence of pain
1-3	Slight or mild pain
4-7	Moderate pain
8-10	Intense or severe pain

Table 3. Scale for gait classification

Scale for gait classification	
0	Normal
1	Occasional claudication
two	Permanent lameness
3	Use of sticks
4	Don't walk

The results were evaluated in the first consultation, six months after cell therapy, in both groups, using the same scales to measure pain intensity (table 2) and classification of gait characteristics, (table 3), from where The lowest numerical values in the evolutionary study indicated the best state of the articulation.

Table 4. OAR grades, according to the Kellgren and Lawrence classification

OAR grades
Grade 0: Normal Grade 1 (Doubtful): Doubtful joint space narrowing. Possible osteophytes. Grade 2 (Light): Possible narrowing of the joint space. Osteophytes. Grade 3 (Moderate): Joint space tightness. Osteophytes. Mild sclerosis. Possible deformity of the ends of the bones. Grade 4 (Severe): Marked narrowing of the joint space. Abundant osteophytes. Severe sclerosis. Deformity of the ends of the bones.

Tomada de Mena and collaborators, 2013 (20)

In this investigation we used the Kellgren and Lawrence classification to evaluate degenerative changes in the joint of the rod (table 3).

2.9 **Clinical response criteria** (25).

The response was medium following the clinical recovery of patients in:

Good: Pain disappears after the 3rd week and continues for 6 months afterwards. Normal ambulation without the need for sticks and which is maintained for 6 months after Regular: Reduction of spontaneous pain or exertion in relation to what existed before the procedure. Occasional claudication

No response: No regular response at all.

2.10 Imagenology

Anteroposterior (AP) and lateral rod X-rays were performed for all patients using internationally established methods (20) before the procedure and six months after the implant.

Response criteria

- Good: Disappearance of degenerative changes, with slight increase in interarticular space and decrease in marginal osteophytes at any time during the year of application of therapy.
- Regular: Decrease in degenerative changes, with a slight increase in interarticular space and decrease in marginal osteophytes at any time during the year of therapy application.
- No answer : No variation in the increase in degenerative changes, interarticular space and marginal osteophytes at any time during the year of therapy application.

2.11 Full response

- Good: Good clinical and radiological response .
- Regular: Regular clinical and radiological response, good clinical and regular radiological response, or vice versa.
- No response : No clinical or radiological response

General and particular data of interest to the investigation are collected in a record created in effect (Annex 1). Data was collected on variable variables such as: clinical symptoms (joint pain, joint soreness, inflammation in the affected wheel, walking disorders, instability

on the wheel, quadriceps hypotrophy, and angular deformities), at the beginning of 6 months, anatomical location of the site of pain, sex, age and global value of the patient according to clinical and radiological recovery.

2.12 . Abandonment criteria

Because of the patient: progression without improvement in symptoms and signs, admission of the patient to another hospital center, death and abandonment of treatment.

2.13 Variables and their operationalization

Variables	1 Type of variable	Indicators

Edad	Quantitative continues	30-39 40-49 50-59 60-69 70-79 +80
Sex	Dichotomous nominal qualitative	-Female -Masculine.
Symptoms y signs	Polytomous nominal qualitative	-Joint pain. - joint chafing. -curdling inflammation affected. - shift to gear. - instability in the wheel. - quadriceps hypotrophy - angular deformities
Anatomical location of the site of pain	Polytomous nominal qualitative	-Rodilla derecha. -Rodilla Izquierda -Bilateral
Criteria for answer	Polytomous nominal qualitative	Buena Regular
Clinic		No response
Gait classification	Discrete polytomous quantitative	The normal 1-Occasional claudication. 2-Permanent lameness 3-Use of sticks 4- Do not walk.
Criteria for response according to scale WOMAC	Polytomous nominal qualitative	Buena Regular No response
Number of patients with adverse effects	Discrete quantitative	Total number of patients who had one or more adverse effects
Adverse effects related to allogeneic platelet lysate	Nominal qualitative	Crisis Vagai Marked pallor Hematoma at the implant site

implantation		
Cost for treat with medication	Quantitative variable to be continued	Calculated in national currency, according to the price of medicines used in conventional treatment, and the production cost of PRP on the average of treatments.
Cost per hospital stay	Quantitative variable to be continued	calculated in national currency, depending on the unit cost of hospital stay and average stay for each treatment
Total cost	Quantitative variable to be continued	Calculated in national currency, given by summarizing previous costs.
Unit cost	Quantitative variable to be continued.	Calculated in national currency, it is calculated by dividing the total cost between the number of patients.
Global valuation	Polytomous nominal qualitative	Buena Regular No response

2.14 Information collection methods

A record sheet was made for each patient with the data obtained from the review of the Individual Clinical Histories (Annex 1).

2.15 Statistical tests

The general and particular data of interest to the investigation was collected in a record made specifically and with them a database was created in Microsoft Excel. Data was collected on variables such as (joint pain, joint soreness, inflammation in the affected wheel, walking disorder, instabilidad in the wheel, hip hypotrophy, and angular deformities), at the beginning of 6 months, anatomical location of the site pain, sex, age and global value of the patient according to clinical and radiological recovery. Descriptive statistical methods are used to summarize qualitative and quantitative variables (absolute and relative percentage frequencies). As is the average and the standard deviation for the estimates. For inferential statistics, the x2 graph was used for the analysis of the association of qualitative variables. To compare clinical symptoms before and after treatment, the McNemar test was used. A pre- and post-implant assessment was carried out using the WOMAC questionnaire (Annex 2) as measuring instruments. The proposed clinical scale consists of five parameters such as: pain, joint function, hip strength, range of movement and the impact of the illness on daily life activities. Each parameter in turn is composed of four aspects with a scoring level differentiated according to its magnitude. The maximum number of points to be achieved is 20 and the minimum is five points. Four questions were generally evaluated ^How much pain do you have?, ^How much stiffness do you feel?, ^How difficult are you in daily tasks? Based on the scale score, differences were established before and after the implant was performed. At every visit, each patient was provided with a form to record the presence of an adverse event. The EPIDAT statistical program version 3.1 was used. The level of significance was $p < 0.05$.

2.16 Economic calculation

In the study group, the cost of handling the platelets to prepare the lysate was calculated, as they were working solely with platelets that, due to their period of conservation, had lost their hemostatic capacity, and were therefore not usable in their usual indications and by blood bank standards they constituted a useful product; also the cost of the equipment with which the lysate is made considering the depreciation of them, which in this case is 30 years and the salary of the staff who work in the studio. The cost of hospitalization was not evaluated because the treatment of this study group is outpatient, the cost of producing platelets in the hospital is 282.04 CUP, per unit of platelets/bag . (Appendix 3).

The control group includes the costs of treatment, with the inclusion of all infiltration material, reagents and used medications that will be used in each patient, plus the cost of the hospital stay in those who need admission, the reason for the price established in it hospital cost of $289.59 MN per day of hospitalization.

2.17 Main limitations of the study

The failure to determine the intraplatelet and serum concentrations of the growth factors that form part of the platelet lysate before its intraarticular administration is recognized as limiting the study, and the failure to perform cartilage biopsies before applying the platelet lysate and after administration is recognized. to determine joint regeneration as the most reliable histological marker to predict healing with confirmation through immunohistochemical marking.

2.18 Ethical aspects

It complied with the principles stipulated in the Declaration of Helsinki (113). Its content in different versions until the current closure includes recommendations for doctors in Biomedical Research in human beings and complies with the principles of medical ethics, the protocol was approved by the Scientific and Ethics Committees for hospital research. All patients were asked for informed consent (Appendix 4), after explaining the characteristics of the study, as well as communicating the possibility of withdrawing from the study at any time they considered it opportune without consequences. Each patient received appropriate information about the objectives, methods, funding sources, possible conflicts of interest, institutional affiliations of the researcher, calculated benefits, predictable risks and inconveniences arising from the investigation. After this is obtained in writing, the person's informed and voluntary consent.

They explain in detail the procedure and the mechanism established in the investigation to form part of each research group.

If the integrity of the patient and the confidentiality of the information were guaranteed at all times, it was impossible to know the personal data of the patients involved in the study. These data are for exclusive use by the team of researchers.

The project received approval from the Cuban Academy of Sciences (ACC), belonging to the Ministry of Science, Technology and the Environment (CITMA).

CHAPTER 3

RESULTS

The characterization of patients according to age showed a predominance of patients over 50 years old (table 5). The average age was 57.6 ± 9.4 years in the group treated with platelet lysate, and 57.1 ± 7.6 years in the group control, means that did not differ significantly (p= 0.5281).

Table 5. Basic characteristics of teaching in the studio according to age

Edad	Platelets allogeneic		Conventional		Total	
	At the.	%	At the.	%	At the.	%
-40	9	1.9	7	1.4	16	3.3
40-49	55	11.3	43	8.9	98	20.2
50-59	79	16.3	61	12.6	140	28.9
≥ 60	129	26.6	102	21.0	231	47.6
Total	272	56.1	213	43.9	485	100.0
Media and DS	57.6 ± 9.4		57.1 ± 7.6			

t = 0.6313 p = 0.5281

Table 6. Distribution of patients according to sex in the study

Sex	Platelets allogeneic		Conventional		Total	
	At the.	%	At the.	%	At the.	%
Masc.	89	18.4	69	14.2	158	32.6
Female.	183	37.7	144	29.7	327	67.4
Total	272	56.1	213	43.9	485	100.0

$X^2 = 0.01$ p = 0.9828

There was an evident predominance of the female sex, in a 3:1 ratio (table 6), with no statistically significant differences in the groups studied.

The distribution of patients according to OAR is shown in (table 7).

Table 7. Distribution of patients according to rod osteoarthritis, Kellgren and Lawrence classification

Degree of OAR	Platelets allogeneic		Conventional		Total	
	At the.	%	At the.	%	At the.	%

0 (normal)	10	3.6	8	3.7	18	3.7
1 (doubtful)	13	4.7	10	4.6	23	4.7
2 (mild)	164	60.2	114	53.5	278	57.3
3 (moderate)	79	29.0	74	34.7	153	31.5
4 (severe)	6	2.2	7	3.2	13	2.6
Total	272	100.0	213	100.0	485	100.0
Media and DS	2.2 ± 0.7		2.3 ± 0.8			

t = 1.4660 p = 0.1413

According to the radiological classification to evaluate rod osteoarthritis (Table 7), 431 patients were between grades 2 and 3; 23, they were dubious and 18 normal. The radiological classification did not have a direct relationship with the pain scale, resulting in 41 patients who had a normal degree or had severe pain. Only 13 grade 4 patients underwent infiltration because this grade is a candidate for rod arthroplasty. There are no significant differences between the treatment groups studied in relation to grades of osteoarthritis or gonarthrosis (p = 0.1413).

When analyzing the presence of comorbidities we can observe that 243 patients had more than one comorbidity, 242 had less than one, which demonstrates the high frequency of association of this condition with other diseases. The most common comorbidities include arterial hypertension, diabetes mellitus, epilepsy; those that accounted for more than 15% of the total number of patients studied (table 8). patients according to type of comorbidity or the presence of a permanent disability factor that prevents blood donation

Comorbidity / Factor	**Number of patients**	**% (N = 485)**
Age > 60	246	50.7
Arterial Hypertension	200	41.2
Diabetes Mellitus	183	37.7
Low weight (less than 50kg)	155	31.9
Epilepsy	58	11.9
Hypothyroidism	10	2.1
Hyperthyroidism	6	1.2
Rheumatoid Arthritis.	4	0.8

Drop	3	0.6

The results regarding initial symptoms and their evaluation over six months in both groups are shown here (table 9).

Table 9. Distribution of frequencies of symptoms and initial and final signs in patients treated with platelet lysate and conventional treatment

y symptoms signs	Allogenic platelets Evaluation.			conventional		
	Home	**to 6 months**	**Mc Nemar***	**Home**	**to 6 months**	**Mc Nemar***
Joint pain	272	52	253.00	213	39	172.01
Chasquido Articulate	61	11	48.02	47	14	31.03
Inflammation of the wheel	86	9	79.01	67	17	48.02
Disruption of it march	234	21	211.00	142	26	114.01
Instability on the wheel	123	55	109.01	96	43	51.02
Hypotrophy of Cuadriceps	25	9	14.06	19	7	10.08
Deformities angular	17	17	0.00	13	13	0.00

***All p values < 0.001**

The symptoms of osteoarthritis were present in both groups, generally appearing overlapping but with one symptom in each patient.

The results that were obtained when evaluating the initial and final symptoms in the groups studied, evidenced significant differences between these moments ($p < 0.03$), which is interpreted as both treatments being effective given the positive modification of these symptoms before and after applying any number of them, with highly significant differences in patients when implanted and lysed ($p < 0.001$).

It can be seen that after 6 months the majority of patients improved, with the exception of 17 who initially presented marked lineage disorders, but most of the pain did not disappear, but there was only a change in their intensity and the disorders remained unchanged. march and the inflammation of

the wheel.

Adverse effects related to the implantation of allogeneic platelet lysate were classified as mild, vagal crisis, marked pallor and hematoma at the implant site

The anatomical location of wheel osteoarthrosis is represented in (table 10).

Table 10. Distribution of patients with wheel osteoarthritis according to anatomical location

Anatomical location	Allogenic platelets		Conventional		Total	
	At the.	%	At the.	%	At the.	%
Rodilla Derecha	65	13.4	50	10.3	115	23.7
Rodilla Izquierda	91	18.8	71	14.6	162	33.4
Bilateral	116	23.9	92	19.0	208	42.9
Total	272	56.1	213	10.3	485	100.0

$X^2 = 0.02$ p = 0.9911

No differences were appreciated (p = 0.9911) regarding the anatomical location of osteoarthritis at the level of the wheel joint. Bilateral involvement is present in 208 cases, which represents 42.9%.

Table 11. Distribution of patients with wheel osteoarthritis according to pain intensity **

Intensity pain	Allogeneic platelets Eva. Initial*	**Eve. to them 6 months	Conventional Eva. Initial*	**Eve. to them 6 months
0-3	27	220	21	105
4-6	76	41	75	72
7-10	169	11	117	36
Total	272	272	213	213
Media and DS	6.8 ± 2.3	2.3 ± 1.8	6.6 ± 2.3	3.9 ± 2.6
t for student	t =148.4318	p = 0.0000	t =131.3507	p = 0.0000

* t = 0.9504 p = 0.3424

** t = 7.9943 p = 0.0000

In the study group, the effective response of the lysate over six months facilitated a marked decrease in the intensity of pain, 220 patients presented the absence of slight joint pain, making the comparison (table 11) resulting in a highly significant difference in the evaluation six months between both groups (p = 0.0000).

Table 12. Frequency distribution regarding gait classification in patients treated with allogeneic platelet lysate and conventional treatment

Classification from the march	Allogenic platelets Initial*	Eva. to them 6 months**	Conventional Initial*	Eva to them 6 months**
0	38	144	30	89
1	56	73	56	56
two	102	34	77	37
3	51	21	29	24
4	25	0	21	7
Total	272	272	213	213
Media and DS	1.9 ± 1.1	0.9 ± 1	1.8 ± 1.1	1.1 ± 1.2
t for student	t = 164.9242 p=0.000		t = 43.7836 p=0.000	

***t = 0.9936 p=0.3209**

1t = 2.0012 p=0.0459

Similar behavior was observed during gear changes (table 12). At the beginning of the study, the total number of patients presented permanent claudication, using sticks or being unable to walk, while after six months, more than three quarters of patients were classified as having normal gait or occasional claudication, which differentiates the treated patients. conventionally, where 7 patients remained without walking.

, including the WOMAC *(The Western Ontario and McMaster Universities Osteoarthritis Index)*. patients before and after implanting platelet lysate (table 13).

Table 13. Distribution of patients according to the WOMAC Scale in pre- and post-treatment evaluation in patients implanted with allogeneic platelet lysate

Aspects to be evaluated.	N =272 Pre-treatment		Posttreatment 6 months	
	Points	Medium	Points	Medium
How much pain is there?	5148	68.6	2002	26.6
How much stiffness do you notice?	4004	53.3	1716	22.8

How difficult is it for daily tasks?	4461	59.4	1430	19

p = 0.019

In the evaluation according to the WOMAC scale, it was found that stiffness had significantly reduced after six months. Likewise, all other evaluated parameters, pain and physical function, improved significantly compared to the initial state; for pain, p = 0.035; for stiffness, p = 0.011; for physical function, one p = 0.034 and the global evaluation one p = 0.019. Table 14. Evaluation of the patient's integral response according to clinical and imaging recovery in the treated groups

Evaluation of it answer	Lysed platelet At the.	%	Treatment Conventional At the.	%	Total	%
Buena	220	80.8	149	69.9	369	76.0
Regular	41	15.0	52	24.4	93	19.1
Sub. Total	261	95.8	201	94.3	462	95.1
No response	11	4.2	12	5.7	23	4.8
Total	272	100.0	213	100.0	485	100.0

$X^2 = 7.8993$ gl=2; p = 0.0193

Significant differences were detected regarding the response between the treatment groups (p= 0.0001). The results were more favorable in the group treated with platelet lysate implant: 95.1% of patients presented a good result in their evolution (of good response but more regular response), with good response predominating in three four parts of the total of them and in the hub it responds in 4.8% of cases. However, 23 patients from the conventional treatment group remained unresponsive (table 14). The comparison between both groups was significant (p= 0.0193).

In the patients of the study group who had a favorable response, there was normal ambulation without the need for rods and it was maintained for six months after that, with the disappearance of degenerative changes, with a slight increase in interarticular space and a decrease in marginal osteophytes (figure 1). The effectiveness of platelet lysate is confirmed through clinical observation of the favorable evolution of the process, in several cases in which reparative phenomena were absent or very slow for very prolonged periods of time. The use of the lysate has a very favorable result, obtaining significant improvements after its intraarticular implant.

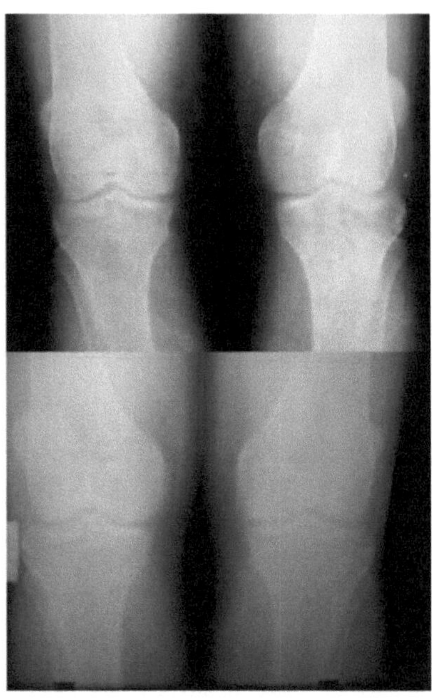

A B

Figure 1. Patient PLC, RAO of 15 years of evolution, **A** : Internal femurotibial joint collapse with severe joint damage, subchondral cysts of the femoral condyles and tibial plates, articular sclerosis, internal femurotibial osteophytes. . **B** : Note after implanting an allogeneic platelet lysate rich in growth factors, recovery of joint space with improvement of joint surfaces and bone density, disappearance of subchondral cysts.

Table 15 shows the costs of treatments carried out in both groups of patients.

Table 15. Average cost per patient across treatment groups in national currency

Treatment	Cost per treatment (MN)	Cost per hospital stay (MN)	Total cost (MN)	Unit cost (MN)
Con Lisado (N=272)	2983.84	0	2983.84	10.97

Conventional (N=213)	32974.32	677.96	33652.28	157.9
Difference	-29990.48	677.96	30668.44	146.93

The cost of drug treatment was $33,652.28 and that of using platelet therapy was $2,983.84 respectively, which represented a saving of $30,668.44.

The unit cost of producing a bag of platelet lysate is minimal when compared to the cost of conventional treatment.

To this advantage we must add that the production of each bag of platelets represents a cost of 282.04 CUP. Which would be the case if this condition were not used for its usual indications for a period of conservation. With the use of platelet lysate, this sum is recovered for each bag used.

CHAPTER 4

DISCUSSION

Regenerative medicine is the one that is responsible for the regeneration and repair of tissues and organs to recover their functionality. Among the regenerative alternatives for osteoarthritis of the rod (RAO), the use of mesenchymal mother cells has been implemented, a technique that is currently in the experimental phase, and is complex and costly in the application of platelet lysate, a procedure of wide use in the current world and object of this evaluation (115).

Platelets are the main source of growth factors in the blood clot, therefore, supra-physiological concentrations of regenerative factors can be achieved by concentrating platelets in a determined volume of plasma and applying them to the site of intraarticular cartilage damage (111).

Osteoarthritis is the most frequently observed joint condition in the adult population of any region of the world, although its prevalence figures vary according to geographic location, different ethnic groups, sex, age of studied populations and the affected joint, for In 2020, it is estimated that the fourth cause of morbidity is more frequent (115), including both sexes affected in a similar proportion, but with symptoms appearing earlier and more severely in women.

In relation to age, there are publications where studies show within their results average age values between 51 and 58.6 years, which is in agreement with this study (110-115).

If it is believed that the increase in the incidence and prevalence of OAR with age is probably due to a cumulative effect due to exposure to various factors and biological changes that occur with aging, such as the thinning of the cartilage, the decrease in muscular strength, changes in propioception and oxidative stress (115). In terms of sex, we can say that it is five times more prevalent in women than in men. There are factors that explain the prevalence of the disease in women such as the higher frequency of obesity, lower muscle tone and greater joint laxity, factors that condition joint instability and favor repetitive microtraumas and therefore joint damage. It is well known that quadriceps weakness is common among patients with RAO, constituting a manifestation of disuse atrophy, which develops because there is discharge from the painful extremity.

Lagojevic in a systematic review on RAO risk factors in older adults, demonstrated that there is an association between the disease and the female sex (OR 1.84, 95% CI 1.32-2.55). Other authors point out that women do not only have a higher frequency of OA than men, but they have a more severe illness (116).

In general, there is a predominance of patients with single or multiple associated comorbidities, which represents 60% of the sample studied. The most frequent chronic illnesses among studied patients were arterial hypertension, diabetes mellitus, epilepsy. Possible explanations for the relationship between OAR and these comorbidities include etiology and physiopathology as well as the result of the biological process of aging, in which different events occur with greater frequency (cartilage degeneration, increased insulin resistance, weight gain, dyslipidemia , oxidative stress) and in this way, they can appear simultaneously, but they no longer need to be interrelated. Perhaps more important than identifying the cause that leads to simultaneity is defining how many of them can influence the health status of patients (117) and prevent them with health education.

Arterial hypertension is recognized as a risk factor for RAO. This could be explained by the presence of oxidative stress that it generates, which plays a preponderant role in the physiopathology of the resulting joint damage.

Chronic inflammatory joint diseases, rheumatoid arthritis, among others, are a recognized cause of secondary RAO, in the literature it refers to producing inflammatory phenomena that lead to joint destruction.

Oxidative stress can be found in the pathophysiological basis of these inflammatory diseases which would justify their association with OAR (118).

It is known that the great affection that produces these affections in the articular cartilage, the main anatomical structure affected in the OAR, where the inflammatory process, metabolic changes and oxidative stress are the main responsible for the destruction of the same, producing additional, deformity, limitation functional and disability that influence the perception of quality of life of patients, this confirms that if from the health and assistance point of view if you want to achieve satisfactory aging, it is necessary to prevent and identify the fragile state early and act on it, with which would be contributing to reducing disability and morbidity in these patients(114).

The most frequent symptoms and signs found were painful and disruptive to gait, both disabling elements, which several authors attribute, in large measure, to anatomical disorders that occur on the wheel, due to ligamentary and osteocartilaginous injuries (119).

On the other hand, its rapid improvement after the implant has been considered to be due to the fact that platelets have analgesic properties secondary to the release of peptides from the protease-activated receptor 4 (PAR-4) (120,121).

Platelets also secrete angiogenic, pro-inflammatory and anti-inflammatory factors. They can interact directly with viruses, bacteria, fungi and protozoa through proteins with direct microbicidal properties that significantly intervene in the defense against pathogenic microorganisms. Among them, peptides called thrombocidins are found, which have antibacterial and antimycotic activity (75).

Coinciding with what was published by Cruz-Sánchez and collaborators (25) in patients with poor alignment, pain persisted, other symptoms such as inflammation and walking disorders after treatment. It is opportune to highlight that in these patients there are favorable changes in the intensity of the symptoms.

If we made a comparison with what was reported by other authors, when analyzing the anatomical location of intraarticular lesions, in a study carried out we found that 65.1% were affected by the right wheel and only 34.8% were affected by the left side, no patients with bilateral affection, these results differ from what was found in our case (122).

From a clinical point of view, pain is the most important symptom and for its explanation there are several theories, one of which is the bad alignment. However, this theory justifies the performance of different surgical re-alignment procedures that on many occasions worsen the patient's symptoms. For this reason, many authors today do not give much value. The author's criteria considers that it is appropriate to perform in these cases corrective osteotomy (procedure or surgical technique suitable for correcting the deformity) and subsequently perform the implant.

Another theory that relates to pain is tissue homeostasis, which is defined as the normal metabolic behavior of biological structures at the cellular and molecular level. The presence of pain reflects the loss of tissue homeostasis due to the presence of biomechanical and biochemical situations (123).

The tendency towards better pain, when we analyze the post-implant EVA, confirms the anti-inflammatory and analgesic effect of platelet factors, which also allows the patient's clinical recovery.

Since then, there has also been gain in the muscular strength of the hips and notable improvements in the evaluation of physical difficulties, including gait.

Growth factors secreted from platelet alpha granules interact with other molecules that modulate cellular function. In concrete terms, growth factors in direct relation to the extracellular domain of transmembrane receptors carry out the transduction of secondary signals in the control of subcellular biology (75,88).

The potential benefits of many growth factors have been demonstrated: platelet-derived growth factor is a powerful mitogen for connective tissue cells, **transforming growth factor β in soil is morphogenetic and** is also strongly implicated in it. collagen synthesis; The type I insulin-dependent growth factor is fundamental for cell survival, growth and metabolism; and the cooperation of the actions of the vascular endothelial growth factor (VEGF) and the hepatocyte growth factor induces the proliferation of endothelial cells and helps their migration to vecine tissues (124,125).

Several studies support that these factors are capable of accelerating recovery in cases of involvement of tendons, ligaments, muscles and cartilage (125-127).

The tendons have a low basal metabolic rate and are predisposed to delay healing after an injury. Some investigations have demonstrated that co-cultivation of tenocytes and a preparation rich in growth factors (PRGF; BTI Biotechnology Institute, Vitoria, Spain) increases the proliferation and secretion of the VEGF growth factor and the HGF hepatoocyte. After repeated injection into Achilles tendons obtained from sheep, it was demonstrated that it was capable of improving angiogenesis and decreasing fibrosis. The encouraging results in animals suggest that it is an easy, safe and potentially viable method for clinical application (128).

Gait disturbances are defined by a slowdown in gait speed, instability, changes in the characteristics of the gait (base,

length, ranges of movement) or modification in the synchrony of both, beyond what is expected for age, generating inefficiency for movement and altering the activities of life, after the implant, in the evaluation after six months, the anti-algic stain There was favorable improvement in patients implanted with allogeneic platelet lysate, which was obtained in this study and behaved similar to that described in the literature (16).

On the other hand, no rejection situations were observed and presents an advantage in the ethical-legal aspect of the use of components certified as safe blood, as by properly classifying the donor it is possible to reduce illnesses transmitted by blood or blood components (HIV, hepatitis, syphilis, among others) (73,129).

The limited capacity for self-regeneration of the cartilage and the limitations of current medical treatments for OAR increase the importance of finding possible treatments for degenerative joint changes and verifying their safety and effectiveness. Regenerative treatments with platelet lysate are considered as an alternative capable of regenerating injured tissues and resulting in improving the quality of life of people with RAO and reducing the need to resort to surgical procedures in these patients while undergoing an adequate comprehensive evaluation of implanted patients is added when they are evaluated before and after performing the percutaneous implant (130).

The WOMAC scale is a useful instrument, as well as being a reproducible, economical practical tool, without requiring special studies, which can be applied to different levels of care, identify complications and address them in a timely manner and improve results (132,133) .

Wheel osteoarthritis is believed to be the main cause of disability in a group of chronic illnesses, with direct and indirect costs of high impact on the health economy, which could be even greater in countries on the road to development . In the United States of America, it is estimated that the affected population could go from 40 million in 1995 to 59 million in 2020, even in our country in a study carried out it was recognized that osteomioarticular diseases were the first cause of disability and pensions granted by this concept on top of cardiovascular and neuropsychiatric conditions (7) RAO, rheumatism of soft parts, sacrolumbalgia and even fibromyalgia, are among the entities that most determine labor affectation.

The OAR generates temporary labor disability on the ground, which causes permanent disability. Its prevalence has been underestimated, however in our average well-distributed studies, it is still at 2.7%, which represents a high rate (131).

Another aspect of interest recognized in the literature is that the presence of these chronic injuries causes irregularities in work activity. It has been established that 75% of patients with this illness are at work, and the illness causes work incapacity that varies between two months and a year. Furthermore, this group of patients was jubilee 7.5 years before their corresponding age, which has repercussions on two important aspects: their quality of life and health costs, aspects that are frequently underestimated in daily medical practice (117,131). It is known that one of the most used medications is chondritis sulfate, which is administered orally and 70% of its dose is absorbed in the intestine. The estimated cost of this medicine monthly is 50 dollars (43), requiring the same for years to achieve its chondroprotective effect, as well as the injection of hyaluronate or viscosupplementation and the cost of this modality of treatment can vary from 500 to 1,500 dollars. three to five injections (50).

In this study, the difference in costs between both treatments is very marked. If the relationship between the unitary cost of two therapeutic alternatives is analyzed, it can be seen that the cost of conventional treatment for a patient represents more than five times the importance of using platelet lysate, and could be considered a greater difference if this is the case. that at the time of application of the platelet lysate, the platelets are totally depreciated, which means they have lost their hemostatic capacity and the normal conduct is their desire. Therefore, its recovery as a result represents what in the economic aspect could be considered as a new use of a disposable biological material.

CHAPTER 5

CONCLUSIONS

- The effectiveness of the intraarticular implant with allogeneic platelet lysate in the treatment of osteoarthritis of the rod was confirmed in women with the onset of symptoms around 50 years of age.
- A faster favorable response to the symptoms and signs of the disease with platelet lysate than with conventional therapy was evidenced. No severe adverse reactions were detected with the intraarticular administration of platelet lysate.
- The presence of comorbidities and causes of exclusion for donation was not an impediment to the implant with the use of the allogeneic lysate.
- The evaluation of the response using a scale was adequate, and the reincorporation of patients into their usual work activities was achieved.
- The use of platelet lysate significantly reduces the cost of treatment, because it is outpatient, no medications are used for intraarticular infiltrations and new use is made of disposable biological material.

RECOMMENDATIONS.

1. To carry out a validation of the effectiveness of platelet lysate in the treatment of wheel osteoarthritis through a phase II-III clinical trial.
2. Jointly carrying out an evaluation of the quality of life of patients included in the study is recommended with the clinical trial.

BIBLIOGRAPHIC REFERENCES

1. Mohamed Soliman Ham . Effectiveness of the intra-articular injection of platelet rich plasma in the treatment of patients with primary knee osteoarthritis . The Egyptian Rheumatologist, Volume 37, Issue 3, July 2015, Pages 119-124.

2. Joint cartilage: structure, pathologies and electrical fields as a therapeutic alternative. Revision

of current conceptsThe articular cartilage: Structure and pathologies, and electrical fields as a therapeutic alternative. A review of current concepts. Vol 31, Issue 4 , December 2017, Pages 202-210.

3. Mifune Y, Matsumoto T, Takayama K, Ota S, Li H, Meszaros LB, et al. The effect of platelet-rich plasma on the regenerative therapy of muscle derived stem cells for articular cartilage repair. Osteoarthritis Cartilage. 2013;21(1):175- 85.

4. Molina Matute M, Ojeda Orellana M. Prevalence and factors associated with **overweight and obesity in patients between 40 and 65 years old. Hospital "José Carrasco Arteaga" 2013. Revista Médica HJCA 2015;7:24-7.**

5. Albanese A, Licata ME, Polizzi B, Campisi G. Platelet-rich plasma (PRP) in dental and oral surgery: from the wound healing to bone regeneration. Immun Aging. 2013;10(1):23 .

6. Val CL, López-Torres J, García EM, Navarro MS, Hernández I, Moreno L. Functional situation, self-perception of health and level of physical activity in patients with arthrosis. Aten Primaria. 2017;49(4):224-32.

7. MINSAP. Cuba. National Directorate of Statistics. Health Statistical Yearbook. 2015:17-20. Available at: http://www.one.cu/aec2015.htm. Consulted in May 2016

8. Mifune Y, Matsumoto T, Takayama K, Ota S, Li H, Meszaros LB, et al. The effect of platelet-rich plasma on the regenerative therapy of muscle derived stem cells for articular cartilage repair. Osteoarthritis Cartilage. 2013;21(1):175---85.

9. Anitua E, Prado R, Sánchez M, Orive G. Platelet-RichPlasma: Preparation and Formulation. Oper Tech Orthop.2012;22(1):25---32.

10. Hernández Ramírez P. Historical data on the application of cellular therapy in orthopedics. [Website] [revised 27 February 2016]. Available at: http://www.sld.cu/sitios/medregenerativa /buscar.php?id=23539&iduser=4&id_topic=17

11. Napolitano M, Matera S, Bossio M, Crescibene A, Costabile E, Almolla J, et al. Autologous platelet gel for tissue regeneration in degenerative disorders of the knee. Blood Transfus.2012;10(1):72---7.41.

12. Moreno Raquel, Gaspar Carreno Marisa, Jiménez Torres José, Alonso Herreros José María, Villimar Ana, López Sánchez Piedad. Techniques for obtaining platelet-rich plasma and its use in osteoinductive therapy. FarmHosp. [Internet]. 2015 Jun [cited 2017 Dic 28] ; 39(3): 130-136. Available at:
http://scielo.isciii.es/scielo.php?script=sci_arttext&pid=S1130-63432015000300002&lng=es. http://dx.doi.org/10.7399/fh.2015.39.3.7998 .

13. De La Mata J. Platelet-rich plasma: a new treatment for the rheumatologist? Rheumatol Clinic. mayo de 2013;9(3):166-71.

14. Vaquerizo V, Plasencia MA, Arribas I, Seijas R, Padilla S, Orive G, et al. Comparison of intra-articular injections of plasma rich in growth factors (PRGF-

Endoret) versus Durolanehyaluronic acid in the treatment of patients with symptomatic osteoarthritis: a randomized controlled trial. Arthroscopy.2013;29(10):1635---43 .

15. Simental-Mendía MA, Vílchez-Cavazos JF, Martínez-Rodríguez HG. Platelet-rich plasma in wheel osteoarthrosis: a treatment alternative. Review article. Surgery and Surgeons. 2015 Aug 31;83(4):352-8. BibTeX EndNote RefMan RefWorks

16. Cruz García Yanet, Hernández Cuellar Isabel María, Montero Barceló Bárbara. Clinical epidemiological behavior of osteoarthritis in female patients. Rev Cuba Reumatol [Internet]. 2014 Aug [cited 2016 Jun 30] ; 16(2):.Available:
http://scielo.sld.cu/scielo.php?script=sci arttext&pid=S1817- 59962014000200004&lng=es .

17. Vaca-González JJ, Gutiérrez ML, Garzón-Alvarado DA. Joint cartilage: structure, pathologies and electrical fields as a therapeutic alternative.
Review of current concepts. Colombian Journal of Orthopedics and Traumatology. 2017 Dec 1;31(4):202-10.

18. Rignack Ramírez Liliams, Brizuela Arias Leandro A, Reyes Llerena Gil Alberto, Toledano V Guibert, Hernández Cuellar Zoila Marlene. Preliminary study of patients diagnosed with osteoarthritis in the outpatient care service of the Rheumatology Center. Rev Cuba Reumatol [Internet]. 2013 Dic [cited 2017 Dic 28] ; 15(3): 192-199. Available at: http://scielo.sld.cu/scielo.php?script=sci_arttext&pid=S1817- 59962013000300008&lng=es .

19. Bin Abd Razak HR1,Heng HY, Cheng KY, Mitra AK. Correlation between radiographic andthroscopic findings in Asian osteoarthritic knees. J Orthop Surg (Hong Kong). 2014;22(2):155-7.

20. Mena Pérez R, Fernández Delgado N, Dinza Zamora L. Use of platelet lysate in rod arthrosis. Rev haban cienc méd [revista en la Internet]. 2013 Sep [cited 14 enero 2014];12(3):374-86. Available at: http://scielo.sld.cu/scielo.php?pid=S1729-519X2013000300010&script=sci_arttext&tlng=en

21. Álvarez López A, Casanova Morote C, García Lorenzo Y, Moras Hernández MA. Rodilla osteoarthritis. Part I review of the theme. Camaguey Medical Archive [Internet]. 2015 [cited 2017 Dic 28];8(4):[approx. 0 p.]. Available at: http://revistaamc.sld.cu/index.php/amc/article/view/3092

22. Gámez Pérez A-. Treatment with mother cells: a new step forward in western Cuba. Cuban Journal of Hematology, Inmunology and Hemotherapy [internet magazine]. 2014 [cited 2016 Jun 30]; 31(1): [approx. 0 p.]. Available at: http://www.revhematologia.sld.cu/index.php/hih/article/view/248

23. Cruz Tamayo F. ¡Don't stop at Ola Regenerativa! Rev Cubana Hematol Inmunol Hemoter.

2013 Mar; 29(1): 1-2.

24. León-Amado L, Díaz-Díaz AJ. Regenerative medicine in Cuba. A revolution that started from the West. Rev Cubana Hematol Inmunol Hemoter. 2013 Sep; 29(3): 213-7.

25. Cruz-Sánchez PM, Gámez-Pérez A, Rodríguez-Orta CA, González Portales Y, López González E, Pérez Mesa D S. et al. Impact of treatment of wheel osteoarthritis with adult mother cells. Rev. Cubana Hematol Inmunol Hemoter 2013; 29(3):272-83.

26. Roemer FW, Eckstein F, Hayashi D, Guermazi A. The role of imaging in osteoarthritis. Best Pract Res Clin Rheumatol. 2014; 28(1):31-60.

27. Medina-Chávez JH. Envelopement of the population and the need for interdisciplinary intervention. Rev Enferm IMSS. 2015; 23 (1): 1-2.

28. Álvarez López Alejandro, Ortega González Carlos, García Lorenzo Yenima, Arias Sifontes Joanka, Ruiz de Villa Suárez Abel. Platelet-rich plasma in patients with gonarthrosis. AMC [Internet]. 2013 Oct [cited 2016 Jun 30]; 17(5): 613-622. Available at: http://scielo.sld.cu/scielo.php?script=sci arttext&pid=S1025- 02552013000500011 &lng=es .

29. Lee KS. Platelet-rich plasma injection. Semin Musculoskelet Radiol. 2013 Feb; 17(1):91-8.

30. Patel S, Dhillon MS, Aggarwal S, Marwaha N, Jain A. Treatment with platelet-rich plasma is more effective than placebo for knee osteoarthritis: a prospective, double-blind, randomized trial. Am J Sports Med. 2013 Feb; 41(2):356-64.

31. Bernstein J, Wolf JM. Autologous blood and platelet-rich plasma injections for enthesopathy of the extensor carpi radialis brevis origin. J Hand Surg Am. 2013 May; 38(5):992-4.

32. Meza-Reyes, G, Aldrete-Velasco, J, Espinosa-Morales, R, Torres-Roldán, F, Díaz-Borjón, A, Robles-San Román, M. Osteoarthrosis: implementation of current diagnostic and therapeutic

algorithms. Revista Médica del Instituto Mexicano del Seguro Social [Internet]. 2017;55(1):67-75. Retrieved from: http://www.redalyc.org/articulo.oa?id=457749297019

33. Gross CE, Hsu AR, Chahal J, Holmes GB Jr. Injectable treatments for noninsertional achilles tendinosis: a systematic review. Foot Ankle Int. 2013 May; 34(5):619-28.

34. Kaux JF, Crielaard JM. Platelet-rich plasma application in the management of chronic tendinopathies. Acta Orthop Belg. 2013 Feb; 79(1):10-5.

35. Martinelli N, Marinozzi A, Carni S, Trovato U, Bianchi A, Denaro V. Platelet-rich plasma injections for chronic plantar fasciitis. Int Orthop. 2013 May; 37(5):839-42.

36. Ramírez Herráiz, E. Economic impact of the use of tumor necrosis factor antagonists in inflammatory arthropathies. Granada: Universidad de Granada, 2016. ---[http://hdl.handle.net/10481/40212] 37. Guzmán López Katherine Natalie, Camas Acero Luis Guillermo, Espinel Núnez Nelson Noé, Ojeda Carpio Adrián Alexander. OverView of regularly used non-steroidal anti-inflammatory drugs in rheumatologic clinical practice prescription. Rev Cuba Reumatol [Internet]. 2017 Apr [cited 2017 Dic 29] ;

19(1): . Available at:

http://scielo.sld.cu/scielo.php?script=sci arttext&pid=S1817- 59962017000100004&lng=es .

38. Gobbi A, Karnatzikos G, Mahajan V, Malchira S. Platelet-rich plasma treatment in symptomatic patients with knee osteoarthritis: preliminary results in a group of active patients. SportsHealth. 2012 Mar; 4(2):162-72.

39. Asay JL, Boyer KA, Andriacchi TP. Repeatability of gait analysis for measuring knee osteoarthritis pain in patients with severe chronic pain. J Orthop Res. 2013 Jul; 31(7):1007-12.

40. Smelter E, Hochberg MC. New treatments for osteoarthritis. Curr Opin Rheumatol. 2013

May; 25(3):310-6.

41. Jordi Monfort, JP, Oren Contreras-Rodríguez, J L-Onaindia, Marina López- Solà, Laura Blanco-Hinojo, Josep Vergés, Marta Herrero, Laura Sánchez, Hector Ortiz, Francisco Montanés, Joan Deus, Pere Benito. Effects of chondroitin sulfate on brain response to painful stimulation in knee osteoarthritis patients. A randomized, double-blind, placebo-controlled functional magnetic resonance imaging study .Medicina Clínica (English Edition), Volume 148, Issue 12, 21 June 2017, Pages 539-547

42. Cala Calvino Leidys, Casas Gross Sandra, Marín Álvarez Tania, Kadel Dunán Cruz Liam. Effectiveness of AliviHo®-rheuma in patients with joint arthrosis. MEDISAN [Internet]. 2017 Mayo [cited 2017 Dic 29] ; 21(5): 564 573. Available at:

http://scielo.sld.cu/scielo.php?script=sci_arttext&pid=S1029- 30192017000500008&lng=es .

43. Mazzocca AD, McCarthy MB, Intravia J, Beitzel K, Apostolakos J, Cote MP, et al. An in vitro evaluation of the anti-inflammatory effects of platelet-rich plasma, ketorolac, and methylprednisolone. Arthroscopy. 2013 Apr; 29(4):675- 83.

44. Marques L, Stessuk T, Cherici I, Junior N, Santos L, Ribeiro Paes J. Platelet-rich plasma (PRP): Methodological aspects and clinical applications. Platelets, Early Online 2015;26(2):101-13. DOI: 10.3109/09537104.2014.881991.

45. Galliera E, Corsi MM, Banfi G. Platelet rich plasma therapy: Inflammatory molecules involved in tissue healing. J Biol Regul Homeost Agents. 2012 Apr- Jun; 26(2 Suppl 1):35-42.

46. Suárez Martín Ricardo, Reyes Pineda Yusimí, López Mantecón Ana Marta, Hernández Muniz Yanileydys, Martínez Larrarte José Pedro. Arthrocentesis and intra and periarticular injections with corticosteroids. Rev Cuba Reumatol [Internet]. 2016 Apr [cited 2017 Dic 29] ; 18(1): 45-61. Available at: http://scielo.sld.cu/scielo.php?script=sci arttext&pid=S1817-

59962016000100008&lng=es .

47. Prosad Bhattacharjee D, Biswas C, Haldar P, Ghosh S, Piplai G, Sankar Rudra J. Efficacy of intraarticular dexamethasone for postoperative analgesia after arthroscopic knee surgery J Anaesthesiol Clin Pharmacol. 2014 Jul- Sep;30(3):387-90. doi: 10.4103/0970-9185.137273

48. Rodrigo-Royo MD, Quero-López JC, Aparicio-Abiol RM, Cía-Blasco P., Baltanás-Rubio P., Acín-Lázaro MP. Efficacy of intraarticular injections of hyaluronic acid for the treatment of osteoarthritis of the rod: results of a series of cases treated in a Unidad del Pain. Rev. Soc. Esp. Pain [Internet]. 2017 Apr [cited 2017 Dic 29] ; 24(2): 74-84.
Available at: http://scielo.isciii.es/scielo.php?script=sci_arttext&pid=S1134-80462017000200074&lng=es .
http://dx.doi.org/10.20986/resed.2016.3485/2016

49. Gutiérrez-Ibarluzea I, Ibargoyen-Roteta N, Benguria-Arrate G, Rada D, Mateos M, Regidor I, Domingo C, González R, Galnares-Cordero L. Sysadoas. Chondroprotectors in the treatment of arthrosis. Ministry of Health, Social Services and Equality. Service for the Evaluation of Sanitary Technologies of the Basque Country; 2013. Health Technology Evaluation Reports: OSTEBA

50. Scott CE, Nutton RW, Biant LC. Lateral compartment osteoarthritis of the knee: Biomechanics and surgical management of end-stage disease. Bone Joint J. 2013 Apr; 95-B (4):436-44.

51. Andriacchi TP, Favre J. The nature of in vivo mechanical signals that influence cartilage health and progression to knee osteoarthritis. Curr Rheumatol Rep. 2014 Nov;16(11):1-8.

52. Morales-Quispe Juan, Suárez Oré César Abraham, Paredes Tafur Claudia, Mendoza Fasabi Vilma, Meza Aguilar Lucero, Colquehuanca Huamani Lumy. Musculoskeletal disorders in recyclers working in Lima

Metropolitan. An. Fac. med. [Internet]. 2016 Oct [cited 2017 Dic 29] ; 77(
4): 357-363. Available at:
http://www.scielo.org.pe/scielo.php?script=sci_arttext&pid=S1025- 55832016000400007&lng=es
.

53. Reginato AM, Riera H, Vera M., et al; Pan-American League of Associations for Rheumatology (PANLAR) Osteoarthritis Study Group. Osteoarthritis in Latin America: Study of Demographic and Clinical Characteristics in 3040 Patients . J Clin Rheumatol 2015; 21 (08) 391-397

54. Wilson Bautista Molano, Daniel Fernández-Avila, Ruth Jiménez, Rosa Cardozo, Andrés Marín, María del Pilar Soler, Olga Gómez, Oscar Ruiz Epidemiological Profile of Colombian Patients With Rheumatoid Arthritis in a Specialized Care Clinic Reumatología Clínica (English Edition), Volume 12 , Issue 6, November-December 2016, Pages 313-318

55. Murawski CD, Hofbauer M, Muller B, Fu FH. Effects of different platelet-rich plasma methods. Am J Sports Med. 2013 Feb; 41(2):NP7.

56. Gálvez-Cano Miguel, Chávez-Jimeno Helver, Aliaga-Diaz Elizabeth. Utility of integral geriatric assessment in the assessment of older adult health. Rev. peru. med. exp. public health [Internet]. 2016 Apr [cited
2017 Dic 29] ; 33(2): 321-327. Available at:
http://www.scielo.org.pe/scielo.php?script=sci_arttext&pid=S1726- 46342016000200018&lng=es
.
http://dx.doi.org/10.17843/rpmesp.2016.332.2204 .

57. Morales Pineiro Sergio, Lennox Warner Darryl, Mata Cuevas Roberto, Morera Estévez Lourdes. Value of roller arthroscopy in older adults.

Medicentro Electrónica [Internet]. 2016 Mar [cited 2017 Dic 29] ; 20(1): 27-37. Available at:

http://scielo.sld.cu/scielo.php?script=sci_arttext&pid=S1029- 30432016000100005&lng=es .

58. Tuan RS, Chen AF, Klatt BA. Cartilage regeneration. J Am Acad Orthop Surg. 2013 may; 21(5): 303-11.

59. VILLAGÓMEZ, Aníbal. Blood platelets. Revista de la Facultad de Ciencias Médicas (Quito), 2017, vol. 1, no 1-4, p. 203-209.

60. MOTTA HERNÁNDEZ, José Wdroo; CARVAJAL CARDOZO, Alexander. Virtual simulation of the classic and cellular coagulation system using Petri nets applying the Virchow test. 2016. Degree Thesis.

61. Vives-Corrons JL, Aguilar-Bascompte JL. Morphological examination of blood cells. JL. Manual of laboratory techniques in hematology. 4th edition. Barcelona, Spain: Editorial Elsevier Masson; 2014. p. 59-93.

62. QUINTANA, A. Moretó, et al. Diseases of primary hemostasis. Vascular purpuras. Platelet diseases. Medicine-Programa de Formación Médica Continuada Accredited, 2016, vol. 12, no 22, p. 1267-1274.

63. By Vasconcelos Torres G, Fernandes Costa IK, da Silva Medeiros RK, Almeida de Oliveira AK, Gomes de Souza AJ, Parreira Mendes FR Characterization of people with venous ulcers in Brazil and Portugal: comparative study. Quarterly electronic nursing magazine. [Internet] 2013 [Cited 2016 Mar 10]; 12(32). Available at:

http://scielo.isciii.es/scielo.php?pid=S1695-61412013000400005&script=sci arttext&tlng=enandothers

64. Osorio-Delgado, Marlon Andrés, Henao-Tamayo, Leydi Johanna, Velásquez-Cock, Jorge Andrés, Canas-Gutierrez, Ana Isabel, Restrepo- Múnera, Luz Marina, Ganán-Rojo, Piedad Felisinda, Zuluaga-Gallego, Robín Octavio, Ortiz -Trujillo, Isabel Cristina, & Castro-Herazo, Cristina Isabel. (2017). Biomedical applications of polymeric biomaterials. DYNA, 84(201), 241-

252. https://dx.doi.org/10.15446/dyna.v84n201.60466

65. Anderson, JM, Future challenges in the in vitro and in vivo evaluation of biomaterial biocompatibility. Regen Biomater, 1, pp. 73-77, 2016. DOI: 10.1093/rb/rbw001.

66. Sheikh, Z., Brooks, P.J., Barzilay, O., et al., Macrophages, foreign body giant cells and their response to implantable biomaterials. Materials (Basel), 8, pp. 5671-5701, 2015. DOI: 10.3390/ma8095269

67. Andia I, Rubio-Azpeitia E, Maffulli N (2015) Platelet-rich plasma modulates the secretion of inflammatory/angiogenic proteins by inflamed tenocytes(2015). Clin Orthop Relat Res 473:1624–1634.

68. F erranti -R amos A ndrea , G arza -G arza G regorio , B átiz -A rmenta J orge , Martínez-Delgado Guillermo, De la Garza-Álvarez Francisco, Martínez-Menchaca Héctor R. et al . Metalloproteinases of the extracellular matrix and their participation in the healing process. UIS Medicines [Internet]. 2017 Aug [cited 2017 Dec 29] ; 30(2): 55-62. Available from http://www.scielo.org.co/scielo.php?script=sci_arttext&pid=S0121-03192017000200055&lng=en . http://dx.doi.org/10.18273/revmed.v30n2- 2017006 .

69. B oyko TV, L ongaker MT, Y ang GP. L aboartory models for the study of normal and pathological wound healing. Plast Reconstr Surg. 2017; 139(3):654- 62.

70. Gould LJ. Topical Collagen=Based Biomaterials for chronic wounds: Rationale and clinical application. Adv Wound Care (New Rochelle). 2016;5(1):19-31.

71. Yun S, Sim E, Goh R, Park J, Han J. Platelet activation: the mechanisms and potential biomarkers. BioMed Research International 2016; 1:1

72. Seijas R, Cuscó X, Sallent A, Serra I, Ares O, Cugat R. Pain in donor si te after BTB -ACL reconstruction with PRGF: a randomized trial. Arch Orthop Trauma Surg 2016; 136(6): 829.

73. Giacomello M, Giacomello A, Mortellaro C, Gallesio G, Mozzati M. Temporomandibular joint disorders treated with articular injection: the effect iveness of plasma rich in growth factors - Endoret. J Craniofac Surg 2015; 26: 709-13.

74. National Institute of Bioengineering and Biomedical Imaging. Fabric engineering and regenerative medicine. IH 2013; 1:1-3.

75. Vaquerizo V, Plasencia M, Arribas I, Seijas R, Padilla S, Orive G.Comparison of intraarticular injections of plasma rich in growth factors

(PRGFEndoret) versus Durolane hyaluronic acid in the treatment of patients with symptomatic osteoarthritis. A randomized controlled trial. Arthrodcopy 2013; 29(10): 1635-43.

76. Morales Ojeda R. Universal Health Coverage. Cuban experience. Cuba Health 2015. International Public Health Convention. La Habana: Editorial Ciencias Médicas; 2015.

77. Bencomo Hernández Antonio A. Platelet derivatives in regenerative medicine. Rev Cubana Hematol Inmunol Hemoter [Internet]. 2012 Dic [cited 2016 Mar 10]; 28(4): [Approx. 1p.]. Available at: http://scielo.sld.cu/scielo.php?script=sci arttext&pid=S0864- 02892012000400001 &lng=es

78. Melians Abreu Silvia María, Núnez López Eloína, Esquivei Hernández Mercedes, Padrino González Maday. Blood as a therapeutic resource from voluntary donation and its social scientific impact. Rev Ciencias Médicas [Internet]. 2017 Feb [cited 2017 Dic 29] ; 21(1): 13-24. Available at: http://scielo.sld.cu/scielo.php?script=sci_arttext&pid=S1561- 31942017000100005&lng=es .

79. Tápanes D, Díaz MD, Martínez J, Tápanes W. The scientific-technical revolution in Medical Sciences in Cuba: since the revolutionary triumph has lasted for several days. Its influence on the health-illness process. Rev Med Electron [Internet]. 2014 [cited 08 Apr 2016]; 36(Suppl-1). Available at: http://scielo.sld.cu/scielo.php?pid=S1684- 18242014000700011 &script=sci arttext

80. Macías Abraham Consuelo. 50 years of work and scientific results of Institute of Hematology and Immunology. Rev Cubana Hematol Inmunol Hemoter [Internet]. 2017 Mar [cited 2017 Dic 29] ; 33(1): 1-7. Available at: http://scielo.sld.cu/scielo.php?script=sci arttext&pid=S0864-02892017000100001 &lng=es .

81. CECMED. Regulation No. M 74-14. Good manufacturing practices for blood establishments. Habana, Cuba: CECMED; 2014.

82. Llano Conrado H, Hernández Santos JR, Tenopala Villegas S, Canseco Aguilar CP and Torres Huerta JC. Effect of platelet-rich plasma and/or growth factors on regeneration and chronic pain associated with intervertebral disc disease. Systematic review. Rev Soc Esp Dolor 2016;23(3):145-153.

83. Barona-Dorado C, González-Regueiro I, Martín-Ares M, Arias-Irimia O, Martínez-González, J. (2014). Efficacy of platelet-rich plasma applied to postextraction retained lower third molar alveoli. A systematic review. Med Oral Patol Oral Cir Bucal, 142-148.

84. Boughner J. (2013). Maintaining perspective on third molar extraction. J. Can. Dent. Assoc, 347-349.

85. Pocaterra A, Caruso S, Bernardi S, et al. Effectiveness of platelet-rich plasma as an adjunctive material to bone graft: a systematic review and meta-analysis of randomized controlled clinical trials. Int J Oral Maxillo-fac Surg. 2016;27:55-70.

86. Martínez Zapata MJ, Martí Caravajal AJ, Solá I, et al. Autologus platelet rich plasma for treating chronic wounds. Cochrane Database Syst Rev. 2016;(5):CD006899.

87. Moraes VY, Lenza M, Tmaoki MJ, et al. Platelet rich therapies for musculoskeletal soft tissue injuries. Cochrane Database Syst Rev.
2014;(4):CD010071.

88. Veitía Cabarrocas F, Arce González MA, Hernández Moreno VJ. Cell therapy in peri-implant disease. First experience in Villa Clara. Medicentro Electrónica. 2013 [cited 22 Mar 2013];17(4). Available at: http://scielo.sld.cu/scielo.php?script=sci_arttext&pid=S1029-30432013000400007

89. Ruggiu A, Ulivi V, Sanguineti F, Cancedda R, Descalzi F. The effect of PlateletLysate on osteoblast proliferation associated with a transient increase of the inflammatory response in bone regeneration. Biomaterials. [Internet]. 2013 [cited 2016 Mar 11]; 34(37): [Approx. 12p.]. Available at:
http://www.sciencedirect.com/science/article/pii/S01 42961213009496

90. Almeida Jéssica Cristina de, Frascino Alexandre Viana M. Bone regeneration in the maxillary sinus. Vital Dentistry [Internet]. 2016 June [cited 2017 Dec 30] ; (24): 29-34. Available from: http://www.scielo.sa.cr/scielo.php?script=sci_arttext&pid=S1659-07752016000100029&lng=en .

91. Scala, A., Lang, NP, Cardoso, LC, Pantani, F., Schweikert, M., Botticelli, D. Sequential healing of the elevated sinus floor after applying autologous bone grafting: an experimental study in minipigs. 2014. Clinic. Oral Impl. Res. 0, / 1-7

92. Escalante Otárola W, Castro Núnez G, Geraldo Vaz L, Carlos Kuga M. Platelet-rich fibrin

(PRF): A therapeutic alternative in dentistry. Rev. Stomatol. Herediana [Internet]. 2016 Jul [cited 2017 Dic 30] ; 26(3): 173-178. Available: http://www.scielo.org.pe/scielo.php?script=sci_arttext&pid=S1019-43552016000300009&lng=es. http://dx.doi.org/10.20453/reh.v26i3.2962

93. Hauser F, Gaydarov N, Badoud I, Vazquez L, Bernard JP, Ammann P. Clinical and histological evaluation of postextraction platelet-rich fibrin socket filling: a prospective randomized controlled study. Dental Implant. 2013; 22:295-303.

94. Robinson Rodríguez Rosa Julia, Ali Pérez Niurka Aurora. Hair biostimulation with platelet-rich plasma against hair loss. MEDISAN [Internet]. 2016 Sep [cited 2017 Dic 30] ; 20(9): 2118-2122. Available at: http://scielo.sld.cu/scielo.php?script=sci_arttext&pid=S1029-30192016000900010&lng=es .

95. Conde Montero E, Fernández Santos ME, Suárez Fernández R. Platelet-rich plasma: applications in dermatology. Actas Dermosifiliogr. 2015; 106 (2): 104-11.

96. Hernández Ramírez Porfirio, Artaza Sánz Heriberto, Aparicio Suárez José Luis, Cruz Tamayo Fernando, Díaz Díaz Antonio Jesús, Fernández Delgado Norma et al. Impact of the regenerative medicine in Angiology. Cuban experience. Rev Cubana Angiol Cir Vasc [Internet]. 2017 Jun [cited 2017 Dic 30] ; 18(1): 3-18. Available at: http://scielo.sld.cu/scielo.php?script=sci arttext&pid=S1682- 00372017000100002&lng=es .

97. Gámez Pérez Anadely, Rodríguez Orta Celia de los A, Arteaga Báez Juan M, Díaz Rodríguez Delia Rosa, Concepción León Ariel, Ricardo Sosa Odalis et al. Growth factors contributed by platelet lysate in the topical treatment of postphlebitic ulcers. Rev Cubana Angiol Cir Vasc [Internet]. 2015 Dic [cited 2017 Dic 30] ; 16(2): 164-174. Available at:

http://scielo.sld.cu/scielo.php?script=sci_arttext&pid=S1682- 00372015000200005&lng=es .

98. _Riestra AC, Alonso-Herreros JM ,Merayo-Lloves J. Platelet-rich plasma on ocular surfacePlatelet-rich plasma on ocular surface. Archivos de la Sociedad Espanola de Oftalmología.Volume 91, Issue 10, October 2016, Pages 475-490

99. Ramírez García Lázara Kenia, Ríos Rodríguez María Elena, Gómez Cabrera Clara Gisela, Rojas Rondón Irene, Gracia Arboleda Juan Carlos. Cutaneous biostimulation using platelet-rich plasma. Rev Cubana Oftalmol [Internet]. 2015 Mar [cited 2017 Dic 30] ; 28(1): . Available at: http://scielo.sld.cu/scielo.php?script=sci_arttext&pid=S0864- 21762015000100011&lng=es .

100. Daphne L, Hutton EM, Moore JM, Grayson G, Grayson WL. Platelet- Derived Growth Factor and Spatiotemporal Cues Induce Development of Vascularized Bone Tissue by Adipose-Derived Stem Cells. Tissue Engineering Part A. [Internet] 2013 [Cited 2016 Mar 10]; 19(17-18): [Approx. 10p]. Available at:
http://www.ncbi.nlm.nih.gov/pmc/articles/pmid/23582144/

101. Franco Mora María del Carmen, Olivares Louhau Ela Maritza, í Pérez Niurka. Regenerative therapy with platelet-rich plasma for
facial rejuvenation. MEDISAN [Internet]. 2015 Nov [cited 2017 Dic 30]
; 19(11): 1353-1358. Available at:
http://scielo.sld.cu/scielo.php?script=sci_arttext&pid=S1029- 30192015001100008&lng=es .

102. Griffiths S, Baraniak PR, Copland IB, Nerem RM, McDevitt TC. Human plateletlysate stimulates high-passage and senescent human multipotent mesenchymal stromal cell growth and rejuvenation in vitro. Cytotherapy, [Internet]. 2013 [Quoted 2016 Mar 10]; 3249(13), 00557-4.

En:

http://www.sciencedirect.com/science/article/pii/S1465324913005574

103. Ruiz-Martínez MA, Morales-Hernández ME. Approach to the treatment of skin aging. Ars Pharm 2015; 56 (4): 183-191.

104. Amable PR, Carias RB, Teixeira MV, da Cruz-Pacheco .I, Corrêa do Amaral RJ, Granjeiro JM et al. Platelet-rich plasma preparation for regenerative medicine: optimization and quantification of cytokines and growth factors. Stem Cell Res Ther 2013; 4 (3): 67.

105. Hernández I., Rossani G., Castro-Sierra R.. Benefits of autologous fibrin adhesive and PRP in rhytidectomy. Cir. plastic. iberolatinoam. [Internet]. 2015 Sep [cited 2017 Dic 30] ; 41(3): 241-258. Available at: http://scielo.isciii.es/scielo.php?script=sci_arttext&pid=S0376-78922015000300005&lng=es . http://dx.doi.org/10.4321/S0376- 78922015000300005

106. Quesada Leyva Lidyce, León Ramentol Cira Cecilia, Fernández Torres Sandra, Nicolau Pestana Elizabeth. Mother cells: a revolution in it regenerative medicine. MEDISAN [Internet]. 2017 Mayo [cited 2017 Dic 30] ; 21(5): 574-581. Available at: http://scielo.sld.cu/scielo.php?script=sci arttext&pid=S1029- 30192017000500009&lng=es .

107. Arce González MA, Hernández Moreno VJ, Penate Gaspar AC. The isolation of mother cells as a scientific-technical service from a transdisciplinary perspective. Medicentro Electrónica. 2013 [cited 12 Ene 2013];17(2). Available at: http://scielo.sld.cu/scielo.php?script=sci arttext&pid=S1029- 30432013000200012

108. Karussis d, Petrou P, Kassis i. Clinical experience with stem cells and other cell therapies in neurological diseases? J neurolSci 2013; 324: 1-9.

109. Naaldijk Y, Jager C, Fabian C, Leovsky C, Bluher A, Rudolph L, et al. Effect of systemic trans-plantation of bone marrow-derived mesenchymal stem cells on neuropathology markers in APP/PS1 Alzheimer mice. neuropathol Appl neurobiol 2016; Feb 26 [Epub ahead of print].

110. Hernández Ramírez P. Tenth anniversary of the fruitful enterprise of regenerative medicine in Cuba. Rev Cubana Hematol Inmunol Hemoter. 2015 Sep;31(3):221-5.

111. Garabano Germán, Lopreite Fernando, del Sel Hernán. Total replacement of the roller in patients under 55 years of age with gonarthrosis: Follow-up for 2 to 13 years. Rev. Asoc. Argent. Ortho. Traumatol. [Internet]. 2017 Jun [cited 2017 Dic 30] ; 82(2): 94-101. Available at: http://www.scielo.org.ar/scielo.php?script=sci arttext&pid=S1852- 74342017000200004&lng=es .

112. Ballester JM, Ballester A, De la Campa J DM, Pérez M, H Hourrutinie B. Procedures for Blood Bank and Transfusion Services. Instituto del Libro.La Habana; 2004.

113. World Medical Association. World Medical Association Declaration of Helsinki: Ethical Principles for Medical Research Involving Human Subjects.

JAMA 2013;310(20):2191-4.Available: http://www.fecicla.org/archivos/articulos/DoH%202013%20ESP.pdf

114. López de Argumedo González de Durana M, Galnares Cordero L. Intra-articular injection of platelet-rich plasma for the treatment of rod arthrosis. Ministry of Health, Social Services and Equality. Service for the Evaluation of Sanitary Technologies of the Basque Country; 2013.

115. Solis Cartas Urbano, Prada Hernández Dinorah Marisabel, Molinero Rodríguez Claudino, de Armas Hernandez Arelys, García González Valia, Hernández Yane Ana. Demographic features in wheel osteoarthritis. Rev Cuba Reumatol [Internet]. 2015 Apr [cited 2016 Jul 14] ;

17(1): 32 39. Available: http://scielo.sld.cu/scielo.php?script=sci arttext&pid=S1817- 59962015000100006&lng=es .

116. Botegoni C., Dei Giudici L., Salvemini S., Chiurazzi E., Bencivenga R., Gigante A. Homologous platelet-rich plasma for the treatment of knee osteoarthritis in selected elderly patients: an open-label, uncontrolled, pilot study. Ther Adv Musculoskelet Dis. 2016 Apr; 8(2): 35—41.

117. Val CL, López-Torres J, García EM, Navarro MS, Hernández I, Moreno L. Functional situation, self-perception of health and level of physical activity in patients with arthrosis. Aten Primaria. 2017;49(4):224-32.

118. . National Institute for Health and Clinical Excellence. Osteoarthritis: care and management in adults. NICE clinical guidelines 117. 2014.

119. Sasaki Eiji, Tsuda E, Yamamoto Y, Iwasaki K, Inoue R, Takahashi I, Ishibashi, **Y. "Serum hyaluronan levels increase with the total number of**

osteoarthritic joints and are strongly associated with the presence of knee and **finger osteoarthritis."** International orthopedics. 2013; 37(5):925-30.

120. Gámez Pérez A, Arteaga Báez JM, Rodríguez Orta CA, López González E, González Cordero F. Advantages of preserved allogeneic platelets in the treatment of lower limb ulcers. Cuban Journal of Hematology, Inmunology and Hemotherapy [internet magazine]. 2013 [cited 24 June 2014];29(1).Available: http://www.revhematologia.sld.cu/index.php/hih/article/view/35/41

121. Álvarez López A, García Lorenzo Y, Ortega González C, García Lorenzo M. Pain anterior de la rodilla. Revista Archivo Médico de Camaguey [internet magazine]. 2014 [cited 2016 Jul 15];14(5):[approx. 0 p.]. Available at: http://revistaamc.sld.cu/index.php/amc/article/view/2118

122. Pacheco Díaz Ernesto A, Arango García Gastón, Jiménez Paneque Rosa, Aballe Hoyos Zenis

A. The intraarticular knee injuries evaluated by arthroscopy, its relationship with clinic and imaging. Rev Cubana Ortop Traumatol [Internet]. 2007 Dic [cited 2016 Jul 15]; 21(2): . Available at: http://scielo.sld.cu/scielo.php?script=sci arttext&pid=S0864-215X2007000200002&lng=es .

123. Jiménez, AR, Fidalgo, AE, Buendía, RA, & Castro, JG Preliminary study with human morphogenetic growth factors in the treatment of rodilla gonarthrosis. Revista de la Sociedad Andaluza de Traumatología y Ortopedia. (2015). 32(1), 63-67.

124. Hutton DL, Moore EM, Gimble JM, Grayson WL. Platelet-derived growth factor and spatiotemporal cues induce development of vascularized bone tissue by adipose-derived stem cells. Tissue Engineering Part A. 2013;19(17- 18):2076-86. doi:10.1089/ten.tea.2012.0752

125. Vaquerizo V, Plasencia M, Arribas I, Seijas R, Padilla S, Orive G, et al. Comparison of intra-articular injections of plasma rich in growth factors (PRGF- Endoret) versus Durolane hyaluronic acid in the treatment of patients with symptomatic osteoarthritis. A randomized controlled trial. Arthrodcopy 2013; 29(10): 1635-43. 8

126. Kadavar G., Demircioglu D., Celik M., Emre T. Effectiveness of plateletrich plasma in the treatment of moderate knee osteoarthritis: a randomized prospective study. J Phys Ther Sci. 2015 Dec;27(12):38637. doi: 10.1589/jpts.27.3863. 15

127. Anitua E, Pelacho B, Prado R, Aguirre J, Sánchez M, Padilla S, et al. Infiltration of plasma rich in growth factors enhances in vivo angiogenesis and improves reperfusion and tissue remodeling after severe hind limb ischemia. Journal of Controlled Release 2015; 202: 31-39.

128. Kutla S, Kukudeveci AA, Elhan AH, Oztuna D, Koc N, Tennant A. Validation of the World Health Organization Disability Assessment Schedule II (WHODAS II) in patients with osteoarthritis. Rev. Reumatol Int. 2011;31:339- 46

129. Contreras A, Reta CB, Torres O, Celis A, Domínguez J. Blood safety in the absence of viral

infections by HBV, HCV and HIV during the serological period of donors.Salud Pública Méx. [Internet] 2011.

[Quoted 2016 Mar 10]; 53(Suppl.1).Availableen: http://www.scielo.org.mx/scielo.php?pid=S0036- 36342011000700004&script=sci arttext

130. Geremicca W, Fonte C, Vecchio S. Blood components for topical use in tissue regeneration: evaluatoin of corneal lesions treated with platelet lysate and considerations on repair mechanisms. Blood Transfusion. [Internet]. 2010 [Quoted 2016 Mar 10]; 8(2): [Approx. 5p.]. Available at: http://www.ncbi.nlm.nih.gov/pmc/articles/PMC2851214/

131. Bernardi M, Albiero E, Alghisi A, Chieregato K, Lievore C, Madeo D, et al. Production of human platelet lysate by use of ultrasound for ex vivo expansion of human bone marrow-derived mesenchymal stromal cells. Cytotherapy. [Internet]. 2013 Aug [cited 2016 Mar 10]; 15(8): [Approx. 9p.]. Available at: http://www.sciencedirect.com/science/article/pii/S146532491300491X

132. Álvarez López Alejandro, García Lorenzo Yenima, Delgado Ceballo Rita María. Clinical scale for patients with primary gonarthrosis: authors' proposal. AMC [Internet]. 2013 Apr [cited 2016 Aug 10] ; 17(2): 129-138. Available at:

http://scielo.sld.cu/scielo.php?script=sci_arttext&pid=S1025- 02552013000200005&lng=es .

133. Escobar A, Vrotsou K, et al. Validation of a reduced functional capacity scale of the WOMAC questionnaire. Gac Sanit. 2011;25(6):513-518. 10

ANNEX 1. Data record sheet (see annex 2 printed in each clinical file))

Reason for Consultation:

History of current illness:

APP:

Previous treatments for the pathology:

Physiotherapy:
Medications: occasional___ sporadic ___ permanent ___
Infiltrations:
Surgical treatments: ___arthroscopy ___ arthrotomy __osteotomy
Others:
Cost of treatment Fees.
Physical examination:
Synovitis:
Valgus deformities - varus
Patellar compression ( )
Joint crepitation ( )
Instability ( )
Joint block ( )
Others:

Radiological assessment:
Right wheel:

Rodilla Izquierda:

Chair:

Shoulder:

Pain rating: 0-3, 4-6,7-10

Gear rating : 0- 1- 2- 3- 4

Diagnostic printing :

Annex 2. WOMAC valuation scale for OAR

The questions from sections **A, B and C** will be asked in a way that shows the continuation.

1. **If you used the "X" according to how you feel:**

Nobody
Pit
Quite
Mucho
Muchísimo
Indicates that **it DOES NOT HAVE PAIN.**

2. **Instructions section A**

The following questions deal with how much **PAIN** you experience in rollers as a result of your arthrosis. (Please mark your answers with an **"X".)**
QUESTION: How painful is it?

1. **While walking on flat land.**

Nobody

Pit
Quite
Mucho
Muchísimo
2. Al climb the lower stairs.
Nobody
Pit
Quite
Mucho
Muchísimo
3. For the night in bed.
Nobody
Pit
Quite
Mucho
Muchísimo
4. The deceased will be sitting there.
Nobody
Pit
Quite
Mucho
Muchísimo
5. Al will be on his feet.
Nobody
Pit
Quite
Mucho
Muchísimo

Instructions section B

The following questions will help you understand how much **RIGIDITY** (in pain) you have noticed on rollers in the last 2 days .

RIGIDITY is a sensation of initial difficulty in moving joints easily.

(Please mark your answers with an "X".)

1. ^How much stiffness do you feel after waking up in the morning?
Nobody
Pool
Quite
Mucha
Muchísima
2. ^How much stiffness do you feel for the rest of the day after sitting, lying down or resting?
Nobody
Pool
Quite
Mucha
Muchísima

Instructions section C

The following questions will help you understand your FUNCTIONAL CAPACITY.

This is your ability to move, move around or take care of yourself.

Indicate how much difficulty you have noticed in the last 2 days when carrying out each of the following activities, as a result of your roller arthrosis.

QUESTION: ^How difficult is it for...?

1. Lower the stairs.
Nobody
Pool
Quite
Mucha
Muchísima
2. Climb the stairs
Nobody
Pool
Quite
Mucha Muchísima
71
3. Get up after sitting.
Nobody
Pool
Quite
Mucha
Muchísima
4. Being on your feet.
Nobody
Pool
Quite
Mucha
Muchísima
5. Squat down to get something out of the ground.
Nobody
Pool
Quite
Mucha
Muchísima
6. Walking through flat terrain.
Nobody
Pool
Quite
Mucha
Muchísima
7. Get in and out of a coach/bus.
Nobody
Pool
Quite
Mucha
Muchísima
8. Go shopping.
Nobody
Pool
Quite
Mucha
Muchísima
9. Put on the media or the pants.
Nobody
Pool
Quite
Mucha

Muchísima
10. Get up from the bed.
Nobody
Pool
Quite
Mucha
Muchísima
11. Remove the media or the calcetines.
Nobody
Pool
Quite
Mucha
Muchísima
12. Being buried in bed.
Nobody
Pool
Quite
Mucha
Muchísima
13. Enter and exit the shower/toilet.
Nobody
Pool
Quite
Mucha
Muchísima
14. Being seated.
Nobody
Pool
Quite
Mucha
Muchísima
15. Sit down and get up from the seat.
Nobody
Pool
Quite
Mucha
Muchísima
16. Carry out heavy household chores.
Nobody
Pool
Quite
Mucha
Muchísima
17. Carry out light household chores.
Nobody
Pool
Quite
Mucha
Muchísima

ANNEX 3. Platelet production cost

Inputs and equipment for the production of platelet concentrate.	Price

	CUP
Lancets-	5.50
Torunda	0.95
Alcohol	0.78/L
Donation	$25.00
Quadruple blood bag	7.64 MN
Rotor 44.26 Initial price	50.20
Table centrifuge Model TDLS-878.00 Initial price	0.66
Cooling centrifuge 1010.3800 Initial price	0.66
Electricity expense.(Production and refrigeration x 72hs	50.20
Hydration	2.75
Seller	3.50
SUMA Pruebas	15.25
Salary expense	15.98
AFT depreciation	13.36
Laboratory rectification	89.61
Total	282.04

ANNEX 4. Informed consent

El (La) que suscribe, ____ y en caso de mis

I freely and voluntarily declare that I have been duly informed by the principal investigator about the procedure to be followed in the investigation. He received verbal information during the interview about the nature, purposes, benefits and alternatives of this investigation, as well as the means with which he considered himself to carry it out and gave my consent to form part of the research demonstration. I have the right to revoke my consent at any time I consider it.

Given to the days of the month of 20.

Patient Name and Surname ___________________________________

Firm _______________________________

Testigo Name and Surname ___________________________________

Firm _______________________________

Investigator Name and Surname ___________________________________

Firm _______________________________

Events.

- **HEMATOLOGIA'2009 Congress: VIII** Latin American Conference on Hematology, Inmunology and Transfusion Medicine. II International Symposium on Regenerative Medicine. III International Hemophilia Workshop. VI Cuban Congress of Hematology. 18-22, May. 2009. Theme Libre. Platelet lysate in postphlebitic ulcers. Application in Cuba.
- Science Day. 14, Enero, 2011. Free theme. Platelet lysate in postphlebitic ulcers
- Research Methodology and Information Management Workshop. 2009. Theme Libre. Efficacy, efficiency and effectiveness of platelet lysate in postphlebitic ulcers.
- VII Methodological Scientific Conference. Pinar del Río. 2009. Theme Libre. Platelet lysate in postphlebitic ulcers. Application in Cuba.
- National Oncohematology Day. San Cristóbal 2009. Theme Libre. Experiences with the use of platelet lysate in postphlebitic ulcers.
- Profesoral Conference and Science and Technique FORUM. San Cristobal. April 16, 2010. Theme Libre. Platelet lysate in postphlebitic ulcers. Application in Cuba.
- XVI Professional and Health Professional Scientific Conference. II Health Convention. June 12, 2010. Theme Libre. Indications for platelet lysate. Application in Cuba.
- National Oncohematology Day. San Cristóbal March 26, 2010. Theme Libre. Platelet lysate in postphlebitic ulcers.
- Nursing Scientific Day. San Cristobal. November 19, 2010. Free Theme. Platelet lysate in postphlebitic ulcers. Application in Cuba.
- X National Congress of Internal Medicine. 25-27 November 2010. Theme Libre. Perspectives on the use of platelet lysate in postphlebitic ulcers.
- Science and Technique Forum, December 20, 2010. Free Theme. Platelet lysate in postphlebitic ulcers. Application in Cuba.
- XVI Science and Technique Forum. 27 days of May 2011. San Cristóbal. Free Theme. Cost-benefit of platelet lysate in postphlebitic ulcers.

- XVI Science and Technique Forum. San Cristobal. People Power. October 27, 2011. Free Theme. Cost-benefit of platelet lysate in postphlebitic ulcers.
- National Day XXX Anniversary. Internal Professional Day. March 2012. Master Conference. Conference. Effectiveness of using platelet lysate in an outpatient setting.
- Profesoral Journey Pinar del Río Medical Sciences University. Effectiveness of the use of platelet lysate in postphlebitic ulcers. 2012
- **Presentation at "Annual Health Award". Provincial Event, May 17,** 2012.
- **Presentation on "Cuban Science Academy Award. February 2013.**
- Provincial Conference of the Cuban Science Union. March/2013.Allogeneic platelet lysate in postphlebitic ulcers.
- **HEMATOLOGIA'2013 Congress: IX Latin American Conference on** Hematology, Inmunology and Transfusion Medicine. III Symposium

  International Regenerative Medicine. IV International Hemophilia Workshop. VII Cuban Congress of Hematology. 24-29, May. 2013. Theme Libre. Local application of allogeneic platelet lysate in postphlebitic ulcers.
- I Taller Medicina regenerativa.Sancti Spiritu. Effectiveness of preserved platelets for the outpatient treatment of postphlebitic ulcers. July 2013.
- IHI-CECMED Regenerative Medicine Conference. April 16, 2015
- Regenerative medicine workshop. CIMEQ. October 5-6, 2015

Teaching Activities. (Impartidos)

- Potentialities of Regenerative Medicine in the treatment of ulcers **in lower limbs from 12/8/2008 to 12/12/2008. IOC "Frank País". 40** hours
- Training and training for doctors at Hospital General Abel Santa María Province of Pinar del Río, Hospital Naval Luís Díaz Soto. 2009. Camilo Cienfuegos Hospital. Sancti Spiritu (2013) 80 hours

Recognitions

- o Reconocimiento en el dia de la Ciencia Cubana. 2010. Ministerio Salud Pública.

  Platelet lysate in postphlebitic ulcers.

  Application in Cuba.

- the Forum XVI Relevant Prize for Science and Technique.2011.
- the Premio Anual de la Salud Provincial 2012. Master's Thesis.

  Effectiveness of the use of platelet lysate in postphlebitic ulcers. 2012

- the CITMA Provincial Award. Platelet lysate in postphlebitic ulcers. Application in Cuba.2012
- o Reconocimiento en el dia de la Ciencia Cubana. 2013. Public Health Ministry

- 1st Provincial Scientific Products Fair. Artemisa.2013
- Cuban Academy of Sciences Award. Provincial. Artemisa.2014.
- Technological Innovation Award. Provincial.2014

SCIENTIFIC PRODUCTION BY THE AUTHOR ON THE THEME OF THE THESIS.

1. **Rodríguez Orta C** , Cruz Sánchez P, Gámez Pérez A, Cruz Pérez Y, Blanco Guzmán S, Pérez Lara, et al. Effectiveness of platelet lysate in the treatment of wheel osteoarthritis. Revista Cubana de Reumatología [internet magazine]. 2014 [cited 2016 Feb 29]; 16(3 Suppl. 1): [approx. 7 p.]. Available at: http://www.revreumatologia.sld.cu/index.php/reumatologia/article/view/376

2. Gámez Pérez A, Arteaga Báez JM, **Rodríguez Orta C de los A** , López González E, González Cordero F, Rodríguez E E. Advantages of preserved allogeneic platelets in the treatment of lower limb ulcers. Rev Cubana Hematol Inmunol Hemoter [revista en la Internet]. 2013 Mar [cited 2016 Feb 29] ; 29(1): 104-107. Available at: http://scielo.sld.cu/scielo.php?script=sci arttext&pid=S0864- 02892013000100012&lng=es .

3-Cruz Sánchez PM, Gámez Pérez A, **Rodríguez Orta C de los Á** , González Portales Y, Pérez Blanco M, Arteaga Báez JM et al. Allogeneic platelet lysate in colgajo necrosis. Rev Cubana Hematol Inmunol Hemoter [revista en la Internet]. 2014 Sep [cited 2016 Feb 29] ; 30(3): 288-293. Available at: http://scielo.sld.cu/scielo.php?script=sci arttext&pid=S0864-02892014000300012&lng=es .

4. Gámez Pérez A, Arteaga Báez JM, **Rodríguez Orta C de los A** , Saavedra Martínez N, González Cordero F, Sanabria Negrín JG et al. Local application of platelet lysate to postphlebitic ulcers. Rev Cubana Hematol Inmunol Hemoter [revista en la Internet]. 2012 Dic [cited 2016 Feb 28] ; 28(4): 374 384. Available at: http://scielo.sld.cu/scielo.php?script=sci arttext&pid=S0864- 02892012000400006&lng=es .

5. Gámez Pérez A, **Rodríguez Orta C de los A** , Arteaga Báez Juan M, Díaz Rodríguez DR, Concepción León A, Ricardo Sosa O et al. Growth factors contributed by platelet lysate in the topical treatment of postphlebitic ulcers. Rev Cubana Angiol Cir Vasc [revista en la Internet]. 2015 Dic [cited 2016 Feb 29] ; 16(2): 164-174. Available at: http://scielo.sld.cu/scielo.php?script=sci arttext&pid=S1682- 00372015000200005&lng=es .

6-Pérez Castillo D, Echemendía AL, Munoz Cruz D, **Á de los Rodríguez Orta C** , Piloto Tome KM, Gámez Pérez A. Platelets with therapeutic benefits in lesions of the osteomioarticular system. Rev Cubana Ortop Traumatol [revista en la Internet]. 2015 Jun [cited 2016 Feb 29]; 29(1): 87-93. Available at: http://scielo.sld.cu/scielo.php?script=sci_arttext&pid=S0864-215X2015000100010&lng=es .

7. Gámez Pérez A, Arteaga Báez JM, **Rodríguez Orta C de los A,** González Cordero F, López González E, Ford Revol D, Ricardo Sosa O, Cabrera Fernández. J. Impact of platelet lysate treatment on the recurrence of postphlebitic ulcers. Rev Cub Ang and Cir Vasc [revista en la Internet]. 2016 [cited 2016 Feb 29]; 16(1). Available at: http://bvs.sld.cu/revistas/ang/vol17 1 16/ang10116.htm

EXPERT CRITERIA

Professor DrC. Doctors DrC: José M. Ballester Santovenia

Professor DrC. Lázaro Silva Ramos. II Degree Specialist in Medicine

Internal and Intensive Medicine. Assistant professor.

CHARACTERIZATION OF EXPERTS: (Required requirements)

a) Boast a scientific degree of Dr. in Medical Sciences or Master in Sciences

b) Holds teaching category of Full Professor, Assistant to Consultant

c) Be a 2nd specialist. Grado

d) Having worked for more than 15 years in Teaching or Research.

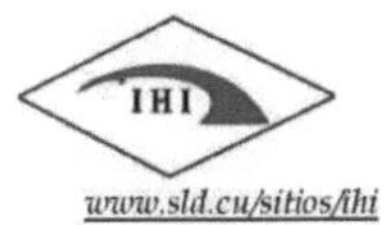

INSTITUTO DE HEMATOLOGIA E INMUNOLOGIA
Apartado Postal 8070, La Habana, CP 10800 CUBA
Tel (537) 6438268, 6438695, Fax (537) 6442334
E-mail ihidir@hemato.sld.cu

La Habana, May 15, 2015
Year 57 of the Revolution

A: SCIENTIFIC GRADES COMMISSION:

SUBJECT: EXPERT CRITERIA

The present thesis work by Dr. Anadely **Gámez Pérez "Effectiveness of the lysate** obtained from allogeneic platelets in the outpatient treatment of **postphlebitic ulcers".**
Refer to the study of the treatment of 90 patients applying platelet lysate to postphlebitic ulcers, which represents the introduction in Cuba of a new method of cellular therapy in the field of Angiology.

It also has methodological and scientific rigor demonstrating the effectiveness and safety in obtaining clinical results. Its scientific impact is given by the possibilities of this new procedure in the healing of ulcerative lesions using platelet lysates preserved as a source of growth factors that induce cell and tissue regeneration.

The effectiveness of the therapeutic procedure corresponds to 70 -80% of treated patients, which allows us to conclude that its introduction and extension in the country constitutes a new therapeutic alternative for these patients suffering from physical and social disability and includes us among the pioneering countries in the successful application of this advanced technique. Its dissemination through publications constitutes the first reports of Cuban literature that addresses the utility of platelet lysate obtained from platelets preserved in postphlebitic ulcers.

For all the above, we consider that this work allows you to opt for the Scientific degree of Doctor in Medical Sciences

Prof. DrC. Consuelo Macías Abraham
PhD in Medical Sciences, professor and researcher.
Full Academic of the Cuban Academy of Sciences
Spec. 2nd. Degree in Immunology
Head of the Department of Immunology
Institute of Hematology and Immunology

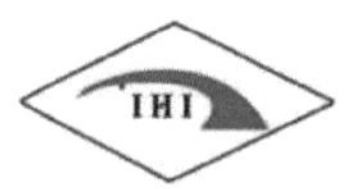

INSTITUTO DE HEMATOLOGIA E INMUNOLOGIA
Apartado Postal 8070, La Habana, CP 10800 CUBA
Tel (537) 6438268, 6438695, Fax (537) 6442334
E-mail ihidir@hemato.sld.cu

www.sld.cu/sitios/ihi

La Habana, May 18, 2013
Year 55 of the Revolution

A: SCIENTIFIC GRADES COMMISSION:

SUBJECT: EXPERT CRITERIA

This is thesis work by Dr. Celia de los Angeles Rodriguez Orta "Effectiveness of allogeneic platelet lysate in the treatment of wheel osteoarthritis". It represents the introduction in Cuba of a new method of cell therapy in the field of Regenerative Medicine.

This work is a new scientific endeavor that is being carried out for the first time in our country. Its scientific impact is given by the possibilities of this new procedure in cell regeneration and joint cartilage recovery from allogeneic platelets as a source of growth factors through a feasible, safe, easy-to-manage and extension method in our National Health System .

It is evident that the effectiveness achieved corresponds to 80% of patients treated by which constitutes a new therapeutic alternative that allows a better quality of life in these sick people and includes us among the few countries that are successfully applying this advanced technique.
The first communication in Cuba on the topic corresponds to the author, results that were exposed at the III International Symposium on Regenerative Medicine at the Hematology Congress 2013.

For all the above, we consider that the job can opt for the Scientific degree of Doctor in Medical Sciences

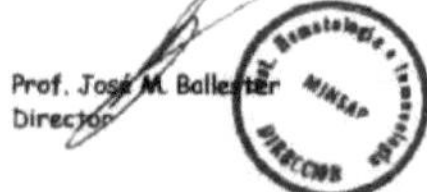

Prof. DrC. José M. Ballester-Santovenia
Doctor in Medical Sciences, professor and researcher.
Full Academic of the Cuban Academy of Sciences
Spec. 2nd. Degree in Hematology
Director of the Institute of Hematology and Immunology

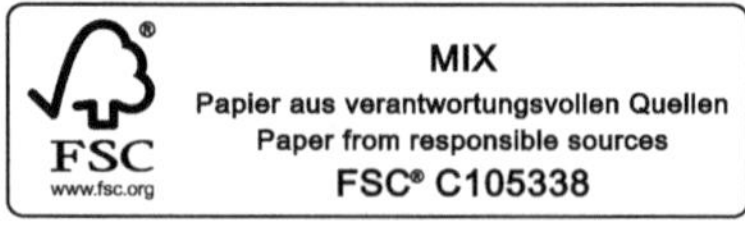

Printed by Books on Demand GmbH, Norderstedt / Germany